# HOW THE
# BODY WORKS

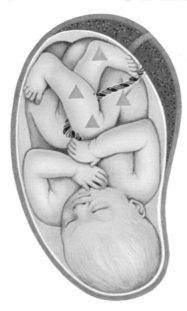

# HOW THE BODY WORKS

## Ron Wilson

## Foreword by Dr Edmund O. Rothschild

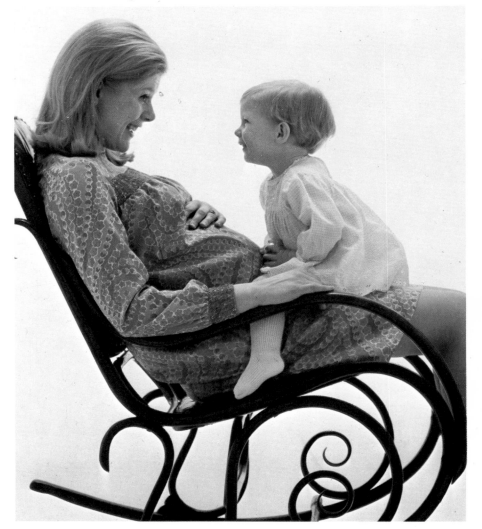

## Larousse and Co. Inc., New York, N.Y.

**Author's note**

I am very grateful to Don Wright, BSc, MSc, Head of the Department of Scientific Studies at the former Kesteven College of Education, and Dr Joan Crawley for reading the manuscript, and making some very valuable suggestions. I am also grateful to Sue Unstead at Ward Lock for her patience and encouragement at all times. I would also express my thanks to Nick Matthews, the local children's librarian, who has been very helpful.

Ron Wilson B.Ed. ACP M.I.Biol.

First Published in United States by
Larousse and Co. Inc.
752 5th Avenue, New York 10036

Published in Great Britain by Ward Lock
Limited, a member of the Pentos Group

ISBN 0–88332–096–7
Library of Congress Catalog Number
78–54036

Printed in Hong Kong

# Contents

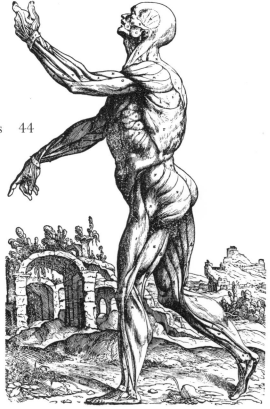

# Foreword

This is a great adventure book, a superior science book, an exciting 'do-it-yourself' book and a basic book about medicine. Once started the reader will want to read it through to the end and then use it again and again as a reference. Written primarily for older children and teen-agers, adults will read it with equal enjoyment.

As a practicing physician I have often wondered why most people know so little about their own bodies. The human body, your body, is an intriguing and fascinating machine. The problem is that most people who understand how it works don't know how to write and therefore make it seem incomprehensible and dull. The challenge is to write about the human body in the exciting and understandable way it deserves and at the same time include important and up-to-date details. This book meets that challenge head on. I have found that the way I best understand how the human body works (and sometimes it doesn't work) is to think in terms of common related examples from the everyday world – I often think in pictures. This book is illustrated throughout and the reader is able to understand complex systems and functions because they are presented in relationship to things he or she already knows or can easily look at.

In this book, you will learn how we all developed from a single almost invisible cell to be born as infants and grow into adults. You will discover how the skeleton and muscles are constructed and how they work to enable us to walk, jump and run. The heart, that incredible pump, and the blood and its circulation will be understandable. Eating, digestion, energy use, elimination of waste, and breathing will become clear to you. You will discover the fascinating details of the senses of feeling, hearing, seeing, tasting and smelling and how they work together with nerves and brain. The complicated functions of speech, coordination and intelligence will not seem as complicated any more. Birth, growth, aging, diseases and their treatment, and hospitals are explored. These and all other functions and structures of your body will become understandable to you and what is more, the whole learning process will be fun.

I personally think this is a rare book which will become a precious one to its owner. I am glad it was written – it is long overdue. You who are about to embark on the adventure of reading it, enjoy and learn – both will be easy and rewarding.

Edmund O. Rothschild M.D., F.A.C.P.

# The cell

Look at the skin on your hands. It consists of millions of individual cells. On the outer surface of the skin or the finger nails these cells happen to be dead, but underneath millions of other cells make up the living tissue of your body.

Cells in other parts of the body are different because they have different jobs to do. If you look at your tongue and the inside of your mouth, you will be observing some of these different types of cell, although you cannot actually see them. Individual cells are so small that they can be seen only under a powerful microscope.

If you look at the section on reproduction (page 62), you will see that you grew originally from just two cells which joined together. It is from those two cells that all the different cells in our bodies have developed. Some cells are larger than others, and each will have its own particular shape.

Next time your mother gets a joint of meat ready for dinner have a look at it before she puts it into the oven.

If it is a leg or shoulder, you will see hard bone surrounded by meat which is muscle and fat. It is likely that you will also see some blood vessels, as well as tissue which holds the muscle to the bone. You can easily distinguish bone, muscles, fat, blood vessels and tissue as each is made up of a different type of cell.

Cells are different because of the various jobs they have to do; at the same time, they all have the same sorts of things in them. It's rather like different types of motor vehicles. Buses, trucks and cars all perform different services and are of various shapes and sizes, yet basically they all have the same sort of parts.

Cells are complicated structures, and we can look only briefly at the main parts. First, each cell has an outer protective membrane. Because it isn't rigid it can change shape easily. It also allows foodstuffs to enter and waste materials to leave.

The largest part of the inside of the cell is made up of cytoplasm, which is rather like a very weak jelly.

Under the microscope a small, darker area can also be seen. This is the nucleus, which has another membrane around it. The nucleus is really the 'control centre' of the cell: it regulates what happens there. If the nucleus dies, then the rest of the cell will also die. The nucleus also carries vital information about such things as the sex of the animal or person, the colour of its hair or eyes, inherited from the time of conception.

The mitochondria are a cell's power houses, converting food into energy, and although cells are very small, some may have more than 500 mitochondria. Cells are working all the while and so they wear out. They are then broken down and replaced by new ones.

*Far left* A magnified section of the tissue from a human nose. Each of the different cells has a special job to do. The larger cells are gland cells which make sticky mucus. This helps to trap dust and dirt in the air which we breathe in. The black dots are nuclei.

*Left* This nerve cell (magnified 2,000 times) is from the spinal cord. The cells receive messages from the brain and pass them to the muscles.

*Opposite* A large cutaway diagrammatic section of a cell showing the main parts. The nucleolus (1) is the central factory of a complex chemical called RNA (Ribonucleic Acid). The nucleus (2) is surrounded by a membrane (3) which is connected to the cell membrane by a channel, the endoplasmic reticulum (4). There are small ribosomes, like dots, along the channel, which make protein. The cell's energy is supplied by the mitochondria (6). The liquids which the cell makes are 'packaged' by the golgi body (9). Waste material is removed by the lysomes (10). There are small spaces –vacuoles (5)–and these either contain fluids or waste materials. Fluid can pass through the cell wall from the outside and is kept in cavities called vesicles (11).

Different types of cells are shown above the large drawing. A a plant cell; B a nerve cell from the brain; C a cell from the lining of the gut and breathing passage; cell D makes up over 90 per cent of the brain and probably nourishes and supports the nerve cells. E a gland cell, putting digestive fluids into the gut; F a muscle cell; G a pigment cell.

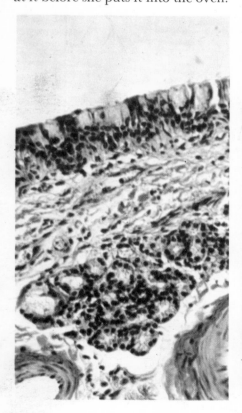

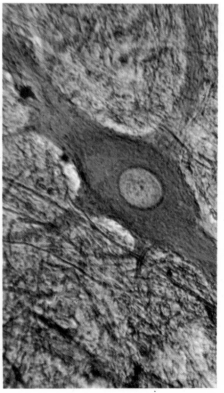

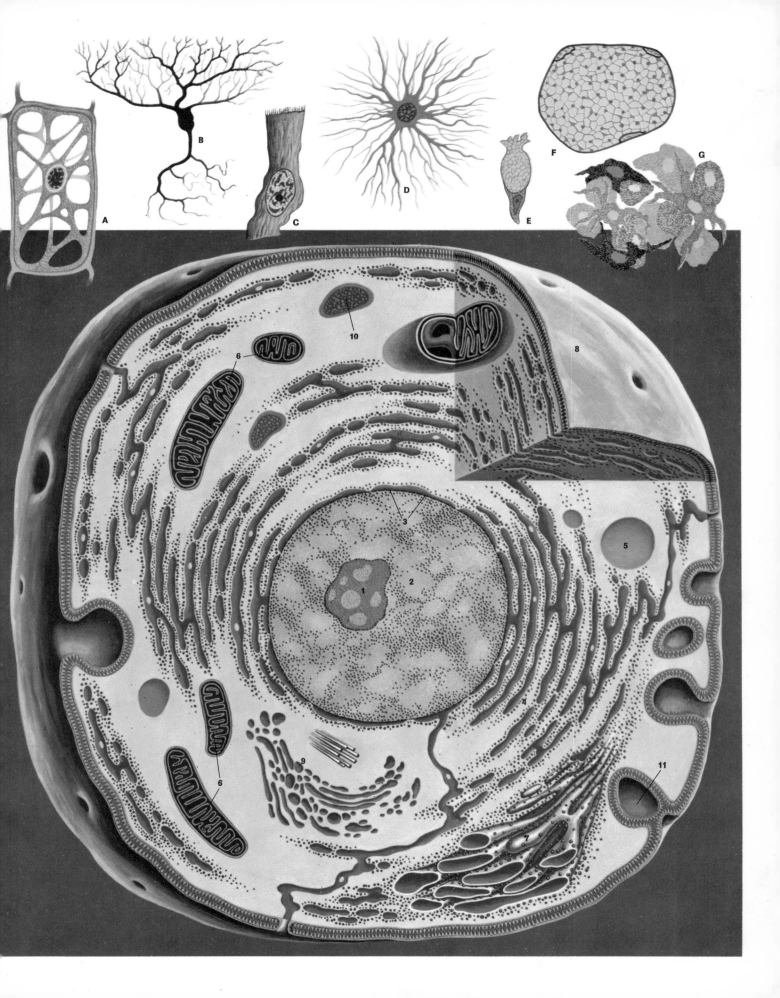

# The skeleton

Have you thought about why you are able to stand up straight and do not collapse in a heap? It is because of the framework of bones inside your body which make up your skeleton. Of these 206 bones which give you your basic shape and support your limbs many are just below the skin. Run your finger from your knee towards your foot. Can you feel the bone just below the surface?

There are some very delicate organs in our bodies, like the brain, the heart and the lungs, and the skeleton also protects these. You can see in the illustration that the bones of the skull are locked together to cover the delicate brain cells. The side view of the skeleton shows that the rib cage sticks out. Attached to the sternum at the front and the bones of the vertebral column—the spine—at the back, the ribs surround the heart and the lungs and so safeguard them. Count the number of ribs and see how many pairs there are.

Our bones need to be strong to support us when we push, pull, lift, run or jump. They also need to be fairly light, otherwise movement would be cumbersome and difficult. Ask your local butcher to cut open a section of bone for you. You will see that the centre is hollow. This bone is dead, but those in your body are living and are supplied with blood and nerves. Your nerves will soon let you know when someone has kicked you!

Long bones in your own body, like the humerus (the upper arm), are also hollow in the centre, although the space is filled with bone marrow. You will see from the illustration of the femur that such bones are wider at the ends, which makes them even stronger. Our bones have a very hard, tough, outer covering consisting of various materials, including calcium phosphate—you will probably have heard people say how important calcium is to the body, particularly in babies. Inside the hard bone casing is another layer called spongy

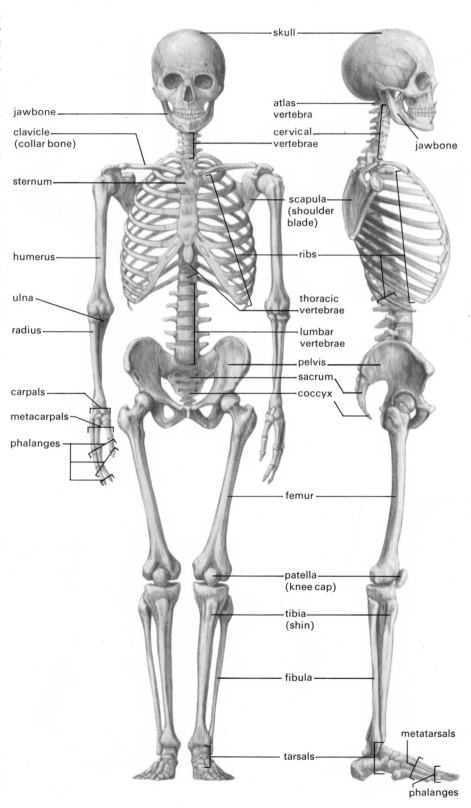

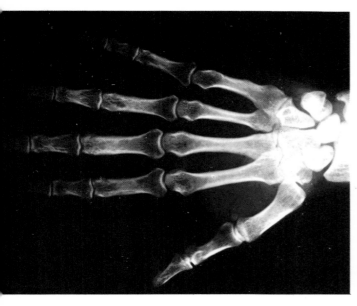

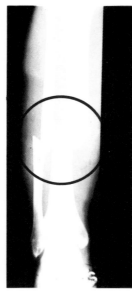

dissolved away each year, and new bone is made, keeping the bones young and supple. However, as people get older, their bone content decreases, until by about the age of 70 only half of the original material is left.

Bones do get broken in spite of their strength. Let us suppose that you have broken a bone. Your doctor cannot be certain exactly what the break is like because he cannot see through the skin, so he will send you for an X-ray. The X-ray machine is able to see through skin and takes a picture of the bone, showing the break. Then your doctor or the hospital staff will know best how to set the bone so that the fractured parts are brought together again. The whole limb will then be covered with plaster of Paris, which will set hard, holding the bones in position.

As soon as a break occurs, a blood clot forms between the two pieces of bone, just as it does if you cut yourself. Reserve cells in the outer lining or sheath of the bone then increase in number, forming a protective covering of fibrous tissues over the break. Within a few days new, young, soft bone cells form at each end of the broken pieces, gradually replacing the tissue. Within three to six weeks the ends of the bone will join up. In the next six to twelve weeks this soft bone will in turn be replaced by harder material. When a bone is set properly, therefore, it will heal completely.

*Opposite* The human skeleton.
*Above left* An X-ray photograph of the normal bone structure in a human hand.
*Above right* An X-ray photograph of a broken human leg. The doctor will have to set it – bring the broken ends together – and then encase the leg in plaster.

bone. This does not mean that it is soft and spongy but describes its sponge-like appearance. It is this material which helps the bone to be both light and strong.

When you were born you were about 50 cm (20 in) long; by the age of 25 you will be, on average, 176 cm (68 in) tall. The bones have grown. How does this happen? In the early stages inside your mother's womb your bones were made of soft cartilage, most being changed to bone before birth. At each end of your bones there is an area of growth cartilage. Here the cells multiply, and the cartilage is gradually replaced with bone. In this way the bones increase in length. About 5 per cent of old bone in our bodies is

- spongy bone
- compact or hard bone
- bone marrow cavity
- bone marrow
- periosteum

*Left* The cutaway section shows the make-up of a femur or thigh-bone. The outside of the bone is made of hard material, with lighter, sponge-like bone inside. The centre of the bone is hollow to make it lighter still.

*Right* A bone looks the same all over, but when viewed under a microscope it is seen to be made up of smaller sections. Like all parts of the body, bone is made of cells. The photomicrograph shows the light areas which are called haversian canals. These will carry blood vessels to the bone. The bone forms in rings around the haversian canals.

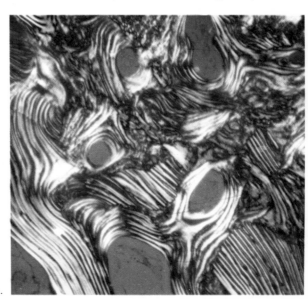

# Muscles and joints

Have you ever wondered exactly how you raise an arm, lift a leg or turn your head round? It is muscles which allow us to perform such actions. The muscles are attached to bones, and we can bend our arms and legs because we have joints where the bones come together. These are called voluntary muscles because we can decide when we want to use them. But we have many so-called involuntary muscles too, over which we have no conscious control. Such muscles control movements of the stomach and intestine; they are even found in blood vessels, and they go on doing their work whether we think about them or not. One vitally important muscle is the cardiac muscle. This is found in the wall of the heart. The heart is a special type of pump which works non-stop throughout our lives. It is not surprising that the muscle is very special, because it has to be extremely strong. Other muscles, like those in our legs, will suffer from fatigue after a while. This does not happen to our heart muscles, although they never stop working.

You will see from the illustrations that the flesh of the body consists of muscles. Like the rest of the body, muscle consists of cells, but these cells are unusual in appearance. Involuntary muscles in the walls between the individual cells have disappeared and they are arranged to form a series of muscle fibres. When viewed under a microscope, these fibres are seen to consist of many thousands of smaller fibres which have a characteristically striped appearance, giving rise to the name striped or striated muscles.

The individual fibres of the voluntary muscles need to work together if we are to move properly, so each has its own nerve supply. A small electrical charge in the muscle makes it contract. Individual fibres contract as much as they can; there is no way of controlling their contraction process. On the other hand, we can control the action of a whole muscle by bringing into use all or only some of the muscle fibres concerned.

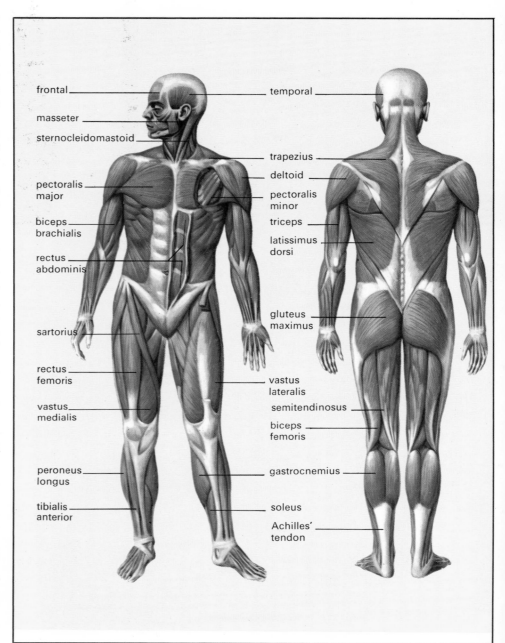

frontal
masseter
sternocleidomastoid
pectoralis major
biceps brachialis
rectus abdominis
sartorius
rectus femoris
vastus medialis
peroneus longus
tibialis anterior

temporal
trapezius
deltoid
pectoralis minor
triceps
latissimus dorsi
gluteus maximus
vastus lateralis
semitendinosus
biceps femoris
gastrocnemius
soleus
Achilles' tendon

Everybody knows that athletes and weight-lifters, as well as keep-fit addicts, have large, well developed muscles. Continuous exercise really does make them grow. We all have the same basic number of fibres in our muscles, but regular exercise of them soon makes them thicker and stronger. The muscles in the arm, for example, can lift a heavier load when they are exercised regularly.

*Above* The illustration of a front view *(left)* and a back view *(right)* of a man shows the main voluntary muscles. The muscles are attached to the bones of the skeleton, and are also known as skeletal muscles. About half the weight of the body consists of these muscles, which work in pairs. When one contracts, the other relaxes. Where muscles are responsible for bending large joints, like that at the elbow, they are known as flexors. Those which straighten the joints are called extensors.

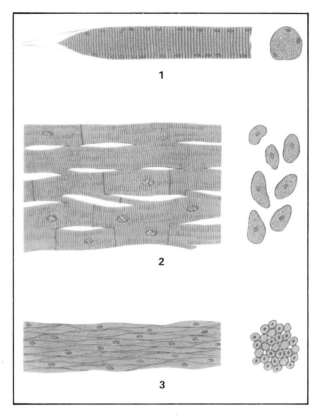

*Left* The three main types of muscles each have different sorts of cell. Long cells are found in striped muscles (1). There are a large number of nuclei in the cells. The cells of the muscle of the heart (cardiac muscle) are much shorter (2). The cells which make up involuntary or smooth muscles (3) are much narrower than either of the other two types.

*Right* Yoga is an excellent method of exercising the muscles and relaxing the body.

*Below* Our arms are very skilfully engineered. The forearm consists of a number of bones, and the muscles are attached to these by tendons. The bones of the lower arm, the radius and ulna, can twist around each other so that we can turn our hands around. Muscles are arranged at various angles so that we can move our arms in different directions.

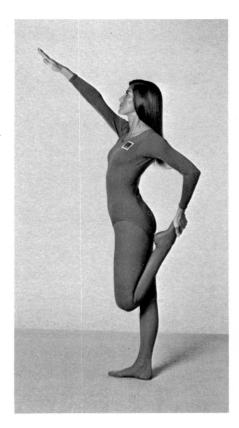

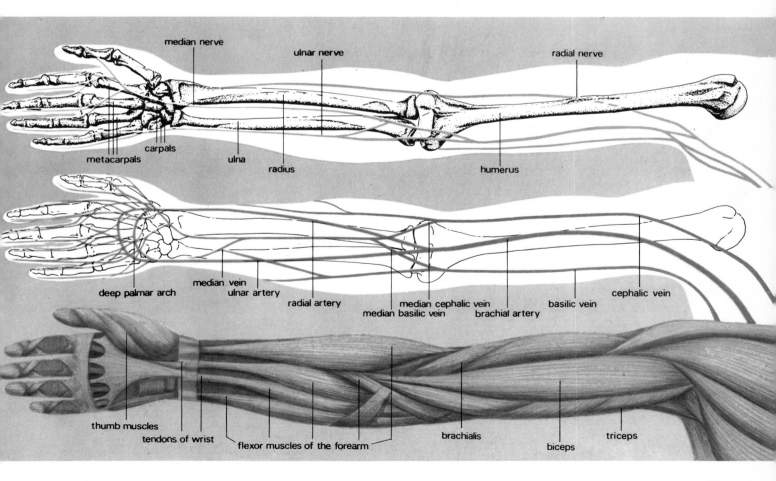

median nerve

ulnar nerve

radial nerve

metacarpals

carpals

ulna

radius

humerus

deep palmar arch

median vein

ulnar artery

radial artery

median cephalic vein

median basilic vein

brachial artery

basilic vein

cephalic vein

thumb muscles

tendons of wrist

flexor muscles of the forearm

brachialis

biceps

triceps

Unless voluntary muscles in our bodies had something to attach themselves to, they would be of little use. So with the help of tendons they are anchored to the bones. At the same time, we would still have great difficulty in moving if, for example, our legs only had one bone. So our arms and legs, hands and feet, shoulders and necks contain a number of bones which allow for bending and twisting movements, each attached to the others by joints. Are all the joints in the body the same? Try moving your shoulder to see how far you can move it. Now move your elbow. Which can you move more freely? The shoulder joint has a greater degree of movement than the elbow because the two joints are different.

There are five different sorts of joint in the body. These are ball and socket, hinge, immovable, pivot and gliding. We have ball and socket joints at the shoulder and at the hips. Make one of your hands into a fist and the other into a cup. Now place the fist in the cup. The fist represents

arm extended

arm flexed

*Far left* The muscles in the arm are attached to the bones. When the muscles at the front of the arm (the biceps) receive signals to contract—shorten—those underneath the arm (the triceps) are instructed to relax. When the arm wants to go down, the opposite happens—the biceps relax and the triceps cotract.
*Left* The voluntary muscles in the body, the ones over which we have some control, have a pulling rather than a pushing action. At the knee the muscles on top of the leg relax (or extend) and those underneath contract. The result is that the leg bends. To straighten the leg the opposite happens.

the ball, and the curled hand the socket. You will see that you can move the fist (ball) quite easily. In the ball and socket joint of the shoulder the ball-shaped top of the humerus fits into a cavity in the scapula or shoulder blade. So that

we can move our arms quite freely at the shoulders the ball fits only into a shallow socket, and dislocated shoulders are quite common. The ball and socket joint at the hip does not allow for so much movement, as you can soon discover for yourself. This is

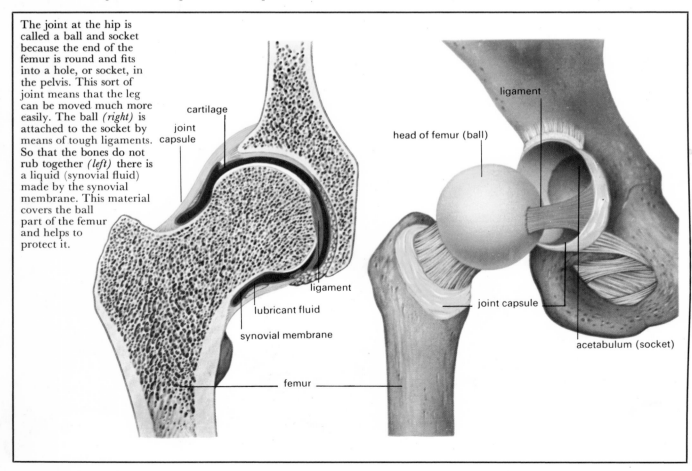

The joint at the hip is called a ball and socket because the end of the femur is round and fits into a hole, or socket, in the pelvis. This sort of joint means that the leg can be moved much more easily. The ball *(right)* is attached to the socket by means of tough ligaments. So that the bones do not rub together *(left)* there is a liquid (synovial fluid) made by the synovial membrane. This material covers the ball part of the femur and helps to protect it.

cartilage

joint capsule

ligament

lubricant fluid

synovial membrane

femur

ligament

head of femur (ball)

joint capsule

acetabulum (socket)

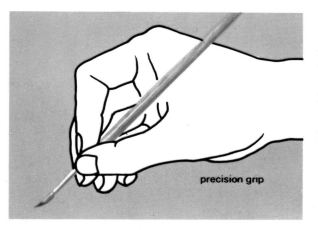

precision grip

With the help of muscles we are able to grip things. Sometimes it might be the fairly thick handle of a cricket bat; sometimes it might be the thin handle of a delicate paintbrush. Here the fingertips come together to hold the paintbrush. The arm will move freely so that the brush can be used.

because the ball-shaped head of the femur bone fits into a far deeper socket in the pelvic girdle than is the case at the shoulder.

In ball and socket joints a tough covering of cartilage covers the bones which helps to prevent wear and tear. The joint is also covered with the synovial membrane. This produces a liquid called the synovial fluid which lubricates the moving parts. Ligaments at the joint also help to straighten it.

We have hinge joints at both the elbow and the knee. These act like hinges and allow us to bend our arms and legs in one direction only.

There are immovable joints between the bones of the skull and in the pelvic girdle. Although your skull bones are now joined, when you were a baby they were separate. As you grew, the bones came together after about eighteen months. If we look at an X-ray photograph of the skull, all we see are faint lines between the bones.

We have a pivot joint at the top of the vertebral column. There are two bones at the top, and a peg on one fits into a hole in the other so that we can move our heads sideways.

Gliding joints are found in the vertebral or spinal column, which is made up of a number of small bones (see page 10). This column of bones acts as a support for the upper half of the body and also allows us to bend and twist, thanks to the gliding and cartilaginous joints. These consist of discs or pads of cartilage between the individual bones of the vertibral column. These discs can be pressed down or twisted slightly, so allowing us to bend or turn the vertebral column.

We have bones, and we have muscles, but what actually makes the joint move? The muscles are attached to bones on either side of the joint. To make the joint move the muscles work in pairs (see page 14). When you straighten your leg, one of the muscles contracts—it gets shorter—while the other relaxes—gets longer. Muscles do not stretch. They exist either at their normal length or they contract. Slowly bend one arm and feel the biceps muscle getting larger as it contracts. Relax the arm again and you can feel the muscle return to its normal length.

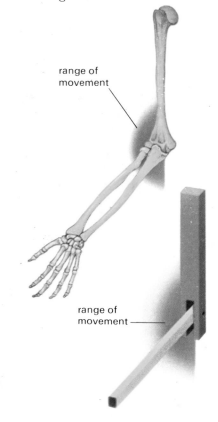

range of movement

range of movement

At the elbow there is a hinge joint, which lets us make only limited movements, when compared to the shoulder joint. The wooden joint *(bottom)* has the same degree of movement as the human one.

Round most of the joints of the body there are several muscles and not just one. This is a good arrangement because it lets us make more than one movement. Try moving your wrist: waggle it about and you will soon see that you can move it in lots of directions, depending on the muscles which are being used.

Take a look at your hand for a minute and then at your fingers in particular. You will soon see that we have a number of joints along each finger. There are lots of small bones in the fingers, and where each meets another there is a joint. At your knuckles you have gliding joints. The bones are flat and smooth and so can move easily over each other. Because the bones are close together, when individual ones move, movement is not very great. When they all move together, quite a lot of movement is possible.

Can you find a hinge joint on your fingers? The one below your nail and the next one down are both hinge joints.

If the muscles become sprained —stretched and torn—they will not relax and contract properly until they have been rested. When this happens, it isn't possible to move the joints without a great deal of pain. Footballers often get sprained ankles, and some tennis players wear bands around their wrists to strengthen them.

15

# The heart

Imagine something like a water pump working for perhaps 70 or more years without attention and without stopping. Impossible, you might say. Yet this is what the heart does in our bodies. You may have seen a sheep's heart in a butcher's shop. Your own heart is very similar. It is really a bag of muscles surrounding four compartments, with a small wall of muscle separating the left-hand side from the right-hand side. The muscles in the heart are very strong because they have to work harder than any of the other muscles in our bodies, pushing the blood to our head and feet. They

stopping the blood from flowing backwards, and at the same time the walls of the top two chambers contract. The valves between the top and bottom compartments open, and the blood is pushed into the ventricles. The valves close, the atria walls relax, and the sides of the bottom two chambers now squeeze, pushing the blood into the large tubes. Look for these names in the diagram. From the left side the blood goes into the aorta, where it will eventually go to all parts of the body. The blood on the right-hand side goes into the pulmonary veins to be taken to the lungs.

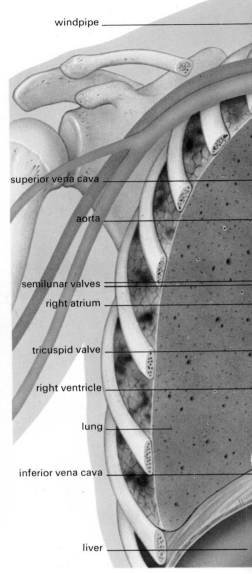

windpipe

superior vena cava

aorta

semilunar valves

right atrium

tricuspid valve

right ventricle

lung

inferior vena cava

liver

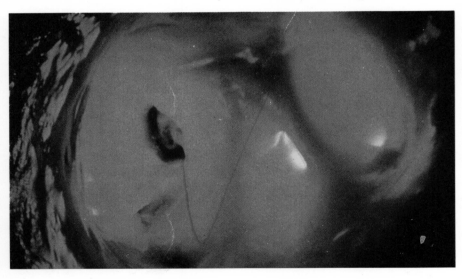

never stop working, except when we die. As the heart is such an essential organ and could easily be damaged, it is protected by the ribs and positioned behind the sternum. When you are fully grown, your heart will weigh about 450 g (1 lb) and be about the size of an adult's clenched fist. At birth it was only 22 g (1 oz). Also, female hearts are slightly smaller than male ones.

Let's see what happens when blood reaches the heart. Blood from the lungs arrives at the left side of the heart. At the same time blood from all other parts of the body will be arriving at the right side. Valves in both sides open to let the blood out of the tubes and into the atria (atrium, singular). The valves close,

*Above* Section through heart muscle. While the heart is working, the thick walls will contract about seventy times a minute – this increases with activity. By beating regularly the blood is pushed through the chambers so that it can be pumped around the body.
*Above right* Cutaway drawing of the heart in relation to the lungs and principal veins and arteries.

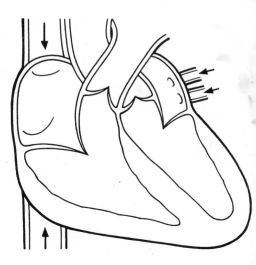

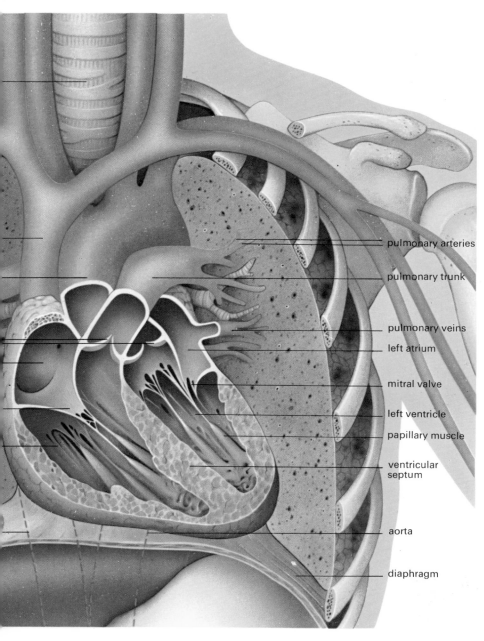

pulmonary arteries

pulmonary trunk

pulmonary veins

left atrium

mitral valve

left ventricle

papillary muscle

ventricular septum

aorta

diaphragm

The heart starts to beat in the embryo forming in the mother's womb, pumping blood around the foetus as it grows and removing waste matter to the placenta. In early foetal life the heart rate is about 65 beats a minute. It rises to about 140 before birth.

The pulse which you can feel at various places in your body, including the wrist, is the heart beat. Let's find out how fast your heart beats. Put your finger—not your thumb, because it has a pulse of its own—on the artery in your arm, just above your wrist. Count the number of beats for half a minute then double the figure. This will be your heart beat. Get your parents and friends to take their pulse and compare theirs with your own. The heart beat is not always the same. Run up and down on the spot for a minute then take your pulse again. Notice how much faster it is. This is because your limbs need more energy in the form of oxygen when you move than when you are resting. The heart must therefore work faster in order to pump the oxygen in your blood to the places where it is needed. Notice too that when you relax the pulse rate takes some time to return to normal while the heart pumps blood carrying oxygen to the respiring tissues.

Although we can control the muscles in our arms when we decide we want to lift something, we cannot control many of the other muscles in the body – the involuntary muscles–including those of the heart. Nerves control how slowly or quickly the heart muscles contract

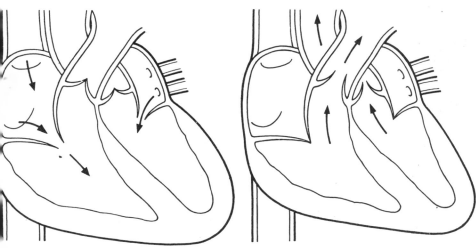

*Left* The diagrams show the cycle of events inside the heart. Blood coming from the body goes into the right atrium. Having come from the body, it does not have much oxygen. At the same time blood rich in oxygen arrives at the left atrium from the lungs. As the atria contract together, they push the blood into the ventricles. The valves close to stop the blood from flowing backwards. The ventricles contract: the blood on the left side goes into the aorta ready to go round the body. Blood in the right ventricle is squeezed out to go to the lungs to pick up oxygen.

and relax and so produce the heart beat. In the right atrium is the natural pacemaker which controls this heart beat. Called the sinu-auricular node, it has muscle and nerve fibres. One set of nerves causes the heart to beat faster: the other set slows the rate down.

If you have a medical examination, the doctor may listen to your heart through a stethoscope. What he or she should hear is a sound like 'lub dub', 'lub dub'. He wants to make sure that the valves in the chambers of the heart are opening and closing properly. He can hear whether any blood is leaking through the valves between one chamber and another between the heart beats. He will be able to find out whether or not there is a hole in the wall of the heart. A doctor's stethoscope is quite expensive, but you could make a simple one for listening to your heart. Try attaching some polythene tubing to a small plastic funnel. Place the funnel on another person's chest (or on your own) and put the tube to your ear. You should be able to hear the beats.

Although we speak of the heart beat, there are in fact two beats involved each time. There is one beat when the atria contract and the valves close and another beat when the ventricles contract and their valves close. If the doctor is not sure about what he hears, he will send the patient to hospital for further tests which might include an electro-cardiograph (ECG). A small machine measures the movements which go on in the heart and records them on a graph. By looking at this the doctor can see if anything is wrong.

Earlier we noticed that the ventricles pumped blood into the arteries. The blood moves along in a series of spurts, and the walls of the arteries, which are elastic, stretch. Between the heart beats they relax, and this helps to move the blood along: this is the blood pressure. When the pressure is either very low or very high, it may be due to disease of the blood vessels or heart.

Sometimes the heart stops beating, and at one time the only way to start it beating again was to cut open the chest and massage the heart. In 1960 an American doctor found that if the chest was massaged about sixty times a minute the heart would often start again. It wasn't necessary to cut open the chest.

One of the modern advances in surgery has been the heart transplant, which Doctor Christian Barnard first carried out successfully in South Africa. Since then surgeons in other countries, including Britain and the United States, have performed similar operations.

If a person has part of his heart damaged, new valves, or perhaps a pacemaker, can be used. But when the heart is badly diseased it will eventually stop, and the person will die. During a transplant a heart-lung machine takes over the normal workings in the body. The diseased heart can them be removed and the new heart put in. When the operation is completed, an electric shock starts the heart beating, and the heart-lung machine can then be disconnected.

In most heart transplants human hearts from people who have died have been used, but sometimes the hearts from monkeys have been transplanted. A 'pick-a-back' idea has also been tried. In this another heart is transplanted, but the diseased heart is not removed. Sometimes the new heart dies. On one or two occasions, when the new heart has stopped beating, the diseased one was found to have started working again. The heart with the defects seems to have had time to recover before the second heart stopped working.

Heart 'murmurs' are quite common, and when a doctor listens to the heart he may hear extra sounds. In many cases these are not dangerous. With modern techniques if a baby is born with a heart defect, it can usually be detected soon after birth. If the defect is very bad, then the baby may soon die, because the heart is unable to carry out its job properly. You have probably heard of babies born with a hole in the heart. The most common cause occurs when there is a hole between the left- and right-hand sides of the heart. In most cases this can be closed with surgery.

When the muscles in the heart do not work regularly, it is possible to install a pacemaker. This small machine will send out electric shocks which make the heart muscles contract at a regular rate instead of erratically.

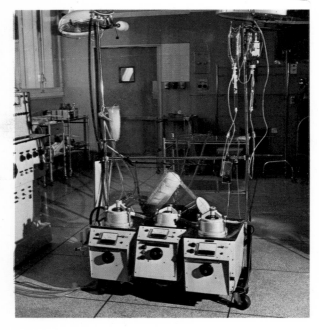

*Left* Heart-lung machines taking over the work of the heart during heart transplant operations. *Opposite (Top)* The body of the person who is to undergo a heart transplant is linked to the heart-lung machine. Blood from the large blood vessels is taken to the heart-lung machine. Carbon dioxide is taken out, and the oxygen replaced. *(Centre)* The diseased heart is taken out and the blood pumped back into an artery situated in the abdomen. *(Bottom)* After the heart has been removed, the replacement heart is put into the body. Once all the blood vessels have been joined, an electric shock will be used to start the heart.

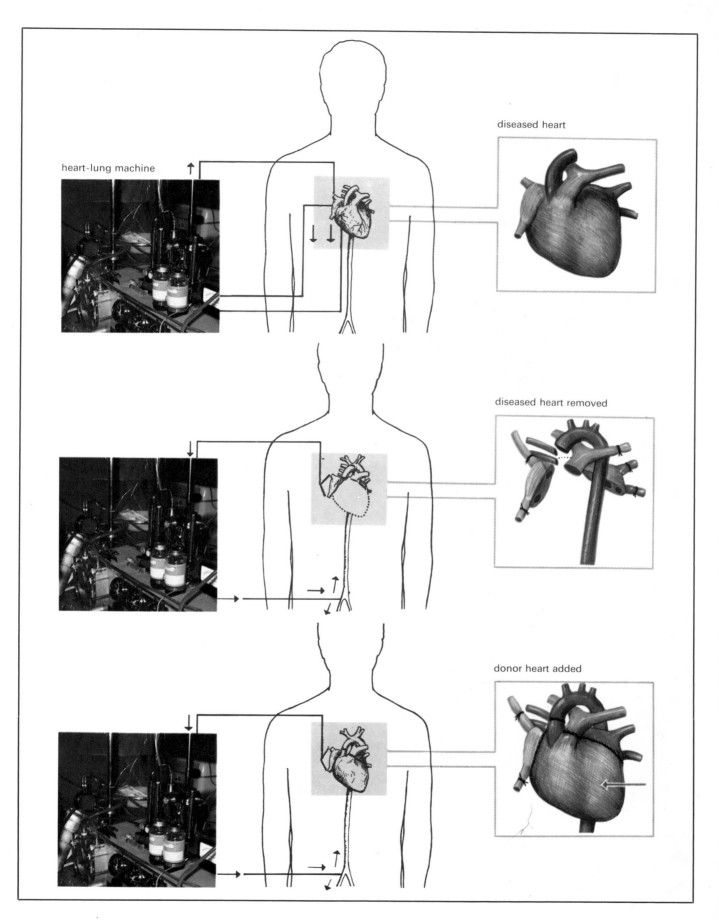

heart-lung machine

diseased heart

diseased heart removed

donor heart added

# The blood

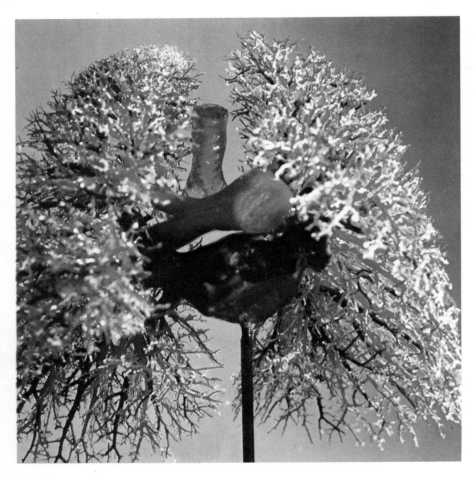

You must have cut yourself at some time or other and seen blood escaping from the wound. Unlike water or many other liquids, blood does not go on escaping from a hole or crack in the skin. It forms a clot beneath which the wound will gradually heal, provided it is not infected.

When blood leaves the body, it looks red because of the colour of some of the cells in it. Blood is made up of two main types of cells. These are the red corpuscles and the white corpuscles, named because of their colour. Each has a very special, although different, job to do. The cells, together with other substances, are carried around the body in a straw-coloured liquid called plasma. The blood has to get to every living cell in the body, and to do this it is pumped by the heart (page 16) through the arteries and veins.

*Above* A model of the blood vessels in the lungs showing how they divide from the larger to the smaller branches. When blood comes to the lungs from the body (blue), it has carbon dioxide in it. When it gives this up, oxygen is taken in. It then flows into the other vessels (red) to go to the heart.
*Right* Red blood cells highly magnified. They carry oxygen attached to the molecules of haemoglobin.

An adult has about 5 litres (11 US pints) of blood. There are more red cells than white ones: about seven hundred red to every white. Blood also carries various minerals, as well as some other cells called platelets. There are waste materials as well.

Every part of our body must have oxygen if we are to survive: the red blood cells are the oxygen carriers. On page 22 you can see how oxygen is taken into the body by the lungs, where it becomes attached to

the red cells and then travels to the heart. From there it is pumped all over the body. The colour of the red corpuscles is due to a substance called haemoglobin, and this can combine with oxygen. At the start of their journeys the red cells have a good supply of oxygen.

Each cell needs a regular supply of oxygen and also produces waste materials. The oxygen is taken to the cell, and waste products from it, by the blood.

The white corpuscles in the blood have another important job to do. Some are known as phagocytes; others as lymphocytes. Phagocyte means 'cell eater'. Such white corpuscles could be compared to soldiers at war, constantly on the lookout for enemies in the body. Some will attack and usually destroy the invaders. Lymphocytes produce chemicals which deal with the poisons produced by bacteria and viruses.

Imagine that you have just cut your finger. All around you, although too small to be seen, are many kinds of bacteria which could make the wound go bad—septic. The white corpuscles will soon be at the scene of the wound dealing with any bacteria. The white cells are not always successful, of course, and infections do occur which have to be treated medically.

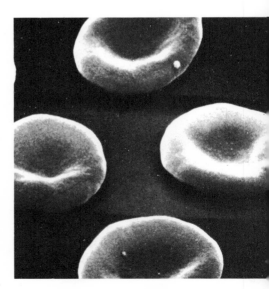

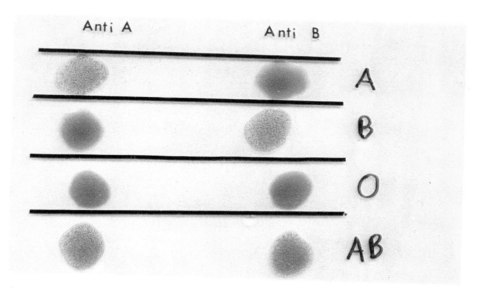

Anti A  Anti B

A
B
O
AB

either in an accident or during an operation. People can be given blood, but it isn't quite as simple as that. Before blood is given, blood samples have to be taken from the person who is going to receive it. These have to be matched with the donor's blood. When the person in need of the blood has been grouped, suitable blood will be obtained from the blood bank.

Each person's blood belongs to one of four main groups, A, B, AB, or O. Because of chemicals in the blood, it is not possible to mix certain groups. People with A group can have blood from A and O. Those in B can have B and O. Those in AB are fortunate because they can

*Above* Blood has to be checked before it can be given to a patient. There are four main blood groups – A, B, AB and O, depending on whether the red cells carry factor A, B, both (AB) or neither (O). Each of the drops of blood has been mixed with an anti-serum to see whether it clots. You will see where the cells have clumped together – Anti-A in A, Anti-B in B, neither in O, both in AB. If the wrong blood was given to a patient, then it would clot, and the person would die.

*Right* The Rh factor was discovered from work carried out on the Rhesus monkey. If anti-Rh serum is added to Rh-positive blood (near diagram), it will clot, but not in the far one.

*Below* Human blood magnified 660 times. A = red blood corpuscles; B = white blood corpuscles; C = a group of platelets. The red corpuscles carry the oxygen, attached to the haemoglobin. The white corpuscles deal with bacteria and viruses which enter the blood, and platelets assist with clotting.

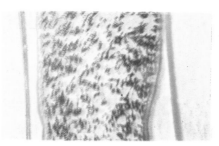

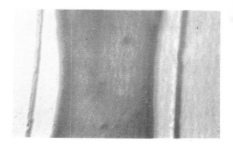

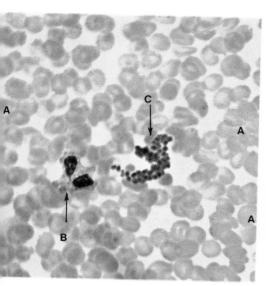

We mentioned earlier that when you cut yourself the blood will soon form a clot and stop flowing from the wound. As a jelly contains gelatine to make it set, so blood has two substances, platelets and fibrin, which perform a similar role. In a wound the platelets cling to each other. The fibrin, which is normally carried in the blood as fibrinogen, starts to become stringy and forms a mesh over the wound, trapping the platelets and corpuscles. Usually this is sufficient to allow the healing process to start, but sometimes with a large cut it is necessary to have stitches to draw the edges of the wound together. There are some unfortunate people who do not have the clotting substance in their blood. This can be very dangerous, because, even with a very small cut, the blood will not clot. A person in his early twenties suffering from this disease, called haemophilia, may have had more than two hundred blood transfusions because of wounds which would not heal; simple injuries could result in death.

Sometimes people do not have enough blood, and some may be lost

have blood from any other group, whereas group O people can have only O blood. If, for example, A was given to B, then chemicals in the blood would make it clot within the blood stream and the patient would die.

You've probably heard of leukaemia as it is quite a common blood disease. Young people suffer from it as well as adults. In acute leukaemia there is a very quick rise in the rate at which the leucocytes – the white cells – are made. There is no certain cure for the disease at the moment, although sufferers often respond to treatment. There are other kinds of leukaemia, and in all cases there is a dangerous increase in one or other of the blood cells. Leukaemia is usually described as 'cancer of the blood'. In spite of much research no one has yet found out why it affects one person and not another.

# Circulation of the blood

The distance from the top of your head to the tip of your toes is probably around 150 cm (5 ft). The cells in your head as well as those in your feet must have blood. The body has to have a system for getting it there. In a water system once the water is collected in a reservoir it has to be sent to everybody. It wouldn't be any use just opening the sluice gates, because the water certainly wouldn't go where it was wanted. Like the water system which needs pipes to supply the consumer, the body needs a system of tubes for circulating the blood. The heart is the pump for pushing the blood round the body.

We have large tubes for taking the blood directly to and from the heart, and smaller tubes for supplying blood to each cell. The large tubes which carry blood with oxygen from the heart are arteries, with the exception of the pulmonary artery which comes from the lungs. The large tubes which go to the heart are veins, with the exception of the pulmonary vein which goes from the heart to the lungs. Capillaries link small arteries and veins, and it is here that the exchange of nutrients and waste materials takes place between tissues and blood.

It is important that the blood keeps circulating all the time. For this reason there are valves in the veins. As the blood pushes, it opens the valves and goes through. The weight of the blood closes the valves behind it. There is still enough pressure in the veins to get the blood back to the heart. The movement of muscles aids the passage of the blood in the veins towards the heart by applying pressure on the veins during muscular contraction. This is known as the venous pump. When someone is inactive or bedridden and their muscles are not being used, the circulation slows down.

Let us see exactly how the blood is circulated. As the atria in the heart relax, blood comes in from the lungs and other parts of the body. With a contraction of the ventricles the blood is pushed out to go to the lungs to get rid of waste, and to the rest of the body to take oxygen.

The arteries branch to form smaller arterioles, which in turn divide to become the smaller capillaries. It is usually these small blood vessels you damage when you cut yourself.

Having done their job by taking blood to every cell, the capillaries join together to form venules, and these then join up to form the veins. The blood will then be taken to the heart. Because arteries have to transport blood all over the body, they have thicker walls than veins.

*Opposite* (1) As the heart relaxes, the blood comes in from the body (blue) and from the lungs (red).
(2) Now the muscles contract, and the blood is squeezed out of the heart to go to the lungs and other parts of the body.
(3) Blood which has been round the body goes to the lungs with its carbon dioxide (blue). As it flows around the alveoli—the small air sacs—it gets rid of its carbon dioxide and takes up oxygen from the air which has been breathed in. The blood (red) is then taken back to the heart.
(4) The blood which flows in the capillaries along the digestive system picks up food. The capillaries join to form the large portal vein, which takes this food to the liver.
(5) Because the cells of the body are so small, the blood system has to split up into very small tubes, the capillaries. These are in contact with the cells.
(6) There are valves in the veins. As blood flows through, it pushes them open. The weight of the blood on the valves then makes them shut.
(7) The body's main blood vessels ensure that the liquid is taken to every part.

*Below* Two X-ray photographs showing the circulation of blood in the head. On the left the arteries can be seen, and on the right the veins.

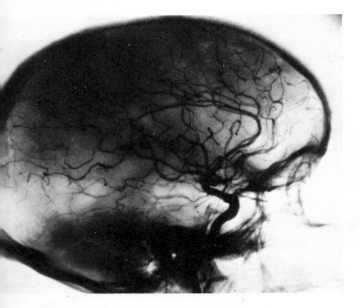
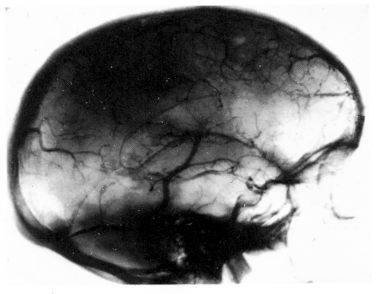

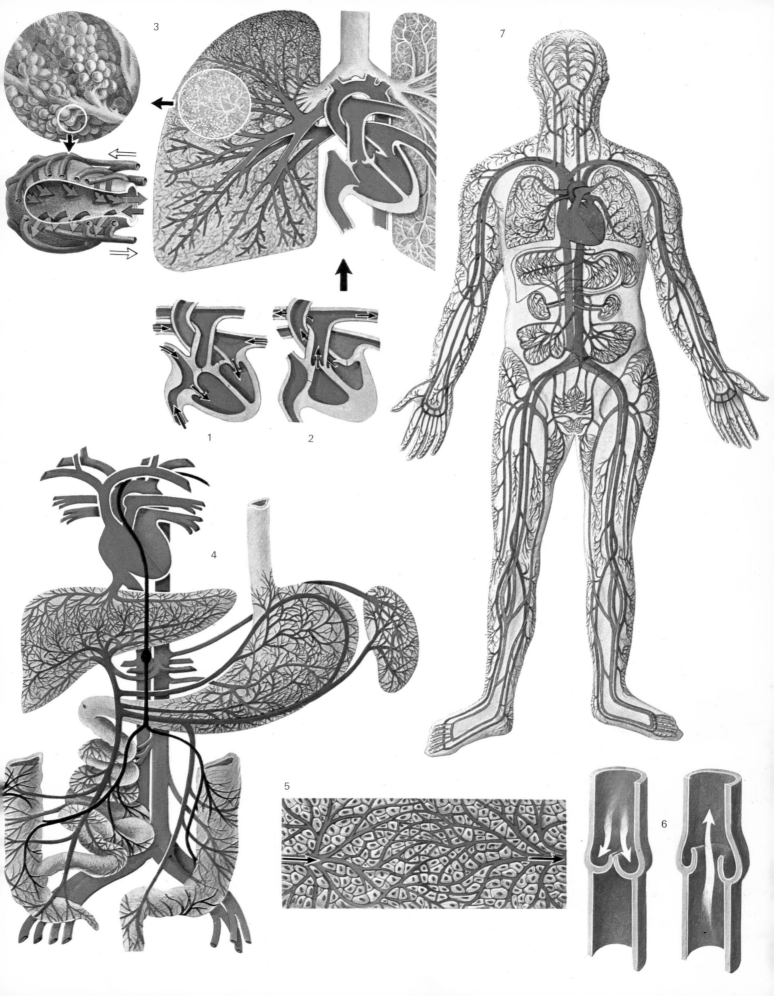

3

7

1

2

4

5

6

# Breathing

The food we digest has to combine with oxygen before it can be converted into energy. The oxygen we need for this purpose is in the air, and we extract from the air as much of it as we require everytime we take a breath. But that is only half the story, for breathing is a two-way process. By breathing in (inspiration) we absorb oxygen into the bloodstream, to be carried to every part of the body which needs it. By breathing out (exhalation) we expel the waste products of the food-into-energy conversion process, mainly carbon dioxide and water, together with those parts of the air not required by the body. The entire process is called respiration, and it is one of the most vital of all bodily functions. It starts at birth and continues right up to the moment of death. People who look as though they are already dead can some-times be revived by artificial respiration, as described in first-aid handbooks; but this needs to be done quickly, for no one can live very long without breathing.

All living creatures breathe. Fishes extract the oxygen in water through their gills. Some insects breathe through their skin. Mammals, which include ourselves, breathe through lungs. Our lungs are situated on either side of the heart, and occupy most of the space in what is called the rib cage. An adult's lungs can contain a surprisingly large quantity of air – during one minute's normal breathing about 6 litres (12 US pints) are inhaled and then exhaled. The passage through which air is taken into the lungs from the nose and mouth, and expelled again with waste products, is the trachea or windpipe. This is strengthened by rings of

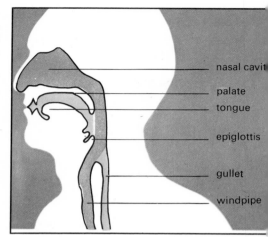

nasal cavit
palate
tongue
epiglottis
gullet
windpipe

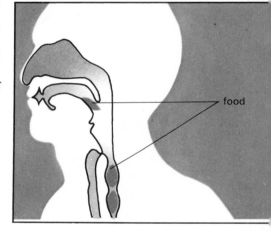

food

tough cartilage so that it remains firm and constantly open. You can feel the trachea in the front of your throat. At the top of the lungs the trachea divides into two tubes called bronchi, one bronchus leading into each lung. The bronchi themselves divide and subdivide into smaller and smaller tubes called bronchioles. These finally terminate in tiny bunches of air sacs, the alveoli. The entire arrangement can be compared to the trunk, branches and foliage of a tree. In appearance a section of healthy human lung is rather sponge-like and pinkish-grey in colour.

When we breathe it may seem that all we do is take in air through nose or mouth, but it is not so simple as that. The whole action commences with our diaphragm, the

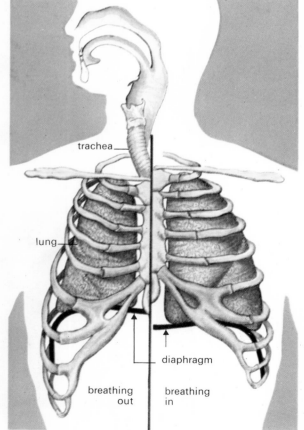

trachea

lung

diaphragm

breathing out    breathing in

*Above right* Cross-section of the head and throat showing the very close connection between mouth, nose, trachea (windpipe) and gullet. The epiglottis plays an essential part in this arrangement, ensuring that food goes down the gullet while only air enters the trachea. In the top diagram the epiglottis is raised, allowing air to pass between nose or mouth and trachea. Below, the epiglottis closes over the top of the trachea while food is swallowed. You cannot breathe and swallow at the same time.

*Left* The lungs inside the rib cage. The part of the drawing to the right of the centre line shows the position of ribs and diaphragm and increased size of the lung as a person breathes in. The left-hand part of the drawing shows the diaphragm and rib position as the person exhales. The lungs draw in and expel air rather like a pair of bellows.

dome-shaped muscular membrane dividing the lungs and heart from the organs or digestion. At the beginning of each breathing action, the diaphragm is lowered, which increases the volume of the lungs from top to bottom. At the same time, other muscles pull the ribs and sternum upwards and outwards, further increasing the space inside the lungs. Only when all this extra lung space has been provided do we actually take in air. In fact, air rushes into the lungs in order to maintain their internal pressure. It travels down the trachea, through the bronchi and bronchioles and finally enters the individual alveoli. It is through the thin tissue of these alveoli that oxygen enters the bloodstream and also that the carbon

*Below* Detail of a single alveolus or air sac. It is here that oxygen from the air passes into the bloodstream via the tiny network of surrounding blood vessels, thence to be circulated round the body. At the same time, carbon dioxide and other waste materials in the blood are returned to the air through the thin, delicate membrane of the alveolus.

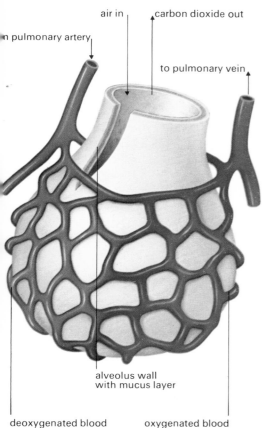

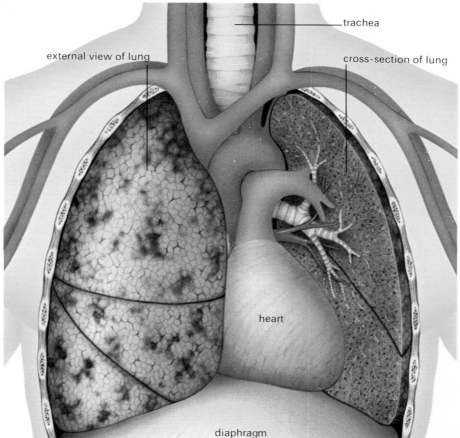

dioxide and other waste products are returned to the air for expulsion. Then, as the diaphragm rises back to its domed position and the ribs contract again, so the air is forced out of the lungs, back up the trachea and out through the nose or mouth.

The breathing process and the rate at which we breathe is one of the many body functions automatically controlled by the brain. When we are resting and not using up much energy, our oxygen needs are relatively small and so our breathing is correspondingly shallow and slow. If we start some strenuous exercise our food-into-energy conversion rate rapidly increases, demanding much more oxygen and therefore a much swifter and deeper rate of breathing. Notice, too, the next time you have been running that you need to keep breathing hard for some time after you have actually stopped. This is because the blood continues to expel the waste products of that exercise through respiration.

The lungs need protection against the many impurities and harmful

*Above* The position of the lungs on either side of the heart. The left-hand lung is shown complete, with its fairly tough but flexible outer casing. The right-hand lung is opened up to reveal the bronchus dividing into smaller bronchioles like the branches of a tree. Note the spongy appearance of the main lung tissue.

organisms in the air. Inside the nose are thousands of minute hairs called cilia which trap many bacteria and particles of dust. This is one reason why it is better to breathe through the nose than the mouth. The trachea and bronchial tubes have more cilia, and also produce a liquid called mucus which keeps them clean and moist and helps to trap further impurities. Mucus and cilia constantly remove dust and other particles by working them gently back towards the mouth or up into the nose. When some really irritating object enters the trachea we start to cough, which pushes the object up into the mouth with the aid of mucus. The nose and trachea also warm the air a little before it enters the lungs.

# We need energy

A car needs fuel to convert into energy to keep it moving. In much the same way our bodies need fuel in the form of food and drink to keep them working.

We can all miss one meal without coming to much harm, because we have a store of food to draw on in emergencies. It is even possible for someone to survive without food (but not without water) for anything up to twelve weeks, though they would probably be seriously ill at the end of that time. In the normal way, however, the quantities and types of foodstuffs our bodies require depends a great deal on how active we might be.

You are probably sitting comfortably reading this book. Hence your body is using up only a fraction of the energy needed by an athlete running in a race. On the other hand, you are consuming some energy all the time. Just by sitting up your muscles need energy to hold your body in position. Now remain as still as possible. Is anything happening in your body? Did you blink? Is your heart still beating? Are you breathing? Of course such actions are taking place, and require energy. Other activities, not so easily detectable, are also taking place all the time, such as the replacement of body cells and, in young people, the actual process of growing. All these things demand energy which comes from food. If you are running, climbing, or kicking a ball you will simply need yet more energy, and therefore more food.

Food can be classified as carbohydrates, fats and proteins. It can also be assessed according to the amount of energy it provides for the body. This energy factor used to be measured in calories (which was a measurement of energy in terms of heat) and is now assessed as joules. In the following list you will see that some foods give us more energy than others.

### ENERGY FOUND IN SOME FOODS

| 1 g of | kilo-joules | 1 g of | kilo-joules |
|---|---|---|---|
| Apple | 1·8 | Cheese | 18·0 |
| Beans, green | 0·5 | Liver | 6·0 |
| | | Margerine | 33·5 |
| Beans, baked | 3·8 | Meat: | |
| | | Beef | 9·0 |
| Biscuits, sweet | 9·2 | Milk | 3·0 |
| Bread | 10·0 | Potatoes, boiled | 3·8 |
| Butter | 33·0 | Sausage, beef | 9·0 |
| Cabbage | 1·0 | | |

Some of the energy from food is used to maintain a body temperature of 37°C (98·4°F). Energy is also required constantly by the muscles, to sustain essential functions like breathing and digestion, and to enable us to move. As food is being broken down in the respiration

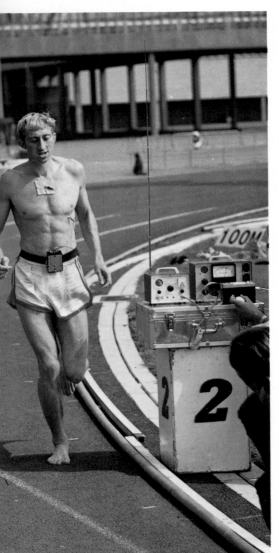

*Left* Scientists want to know what happens to a person's body under 'abnormal' conditions, as well as under 'normal' ones. Here David Hemery, the Olympic medallist, has his body linked up to a recording device. The machine records information about his heart.

*Right* It is possible to find out just how much energy a person needs to stay alive. This is called the Basal Metabolic Rate (BMR). Everyone is different, and each person will have a different BMR. Growing children need more energy than adults. It is clear that as a person gets older less energy is needed. You will also see that it is different for men and women.

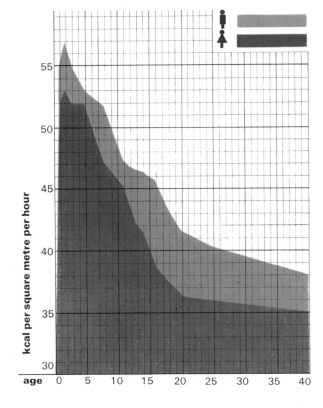

Physiologists use this equipment to measure the rate at which a person takes in oxygen through the lungs. Having measured this, it is then possible to work out how much energy a person uses in, for example, a day. As the patient breathes in and out through the mouthpiece, the pen on the drum records the amount of oxygen taken in. Not all the oxygen we breathe in is used; only about 20 per cent is absorbed by the body.

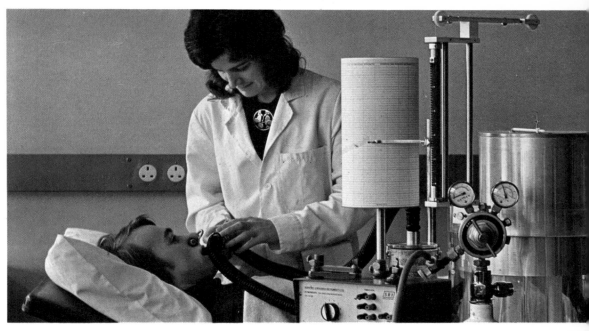

process, oxygen is being consumed, and carbon dioxide given out. The largest amount of carbon dioxide is given out when carbohydrates are being broken down, and the least when fats are being used.

### WHAT'S IN OUR FOOD?

| Food | Carbo-hydrate | Protein | Fats |
|---|---|---|---|
| Apple | 14·0 | 2·0 | 1·0 |
| Banana | 22·0 | 2·3 | 3·0 |
| Beef, lean | 0·0 | 14·0 | 29·0 |
| Bread, brown | 50·0 | 8·5 | 1·3 |
| Butter | 0·0 | 0·5 | 82·5 |
| Cabbage | 3·5 | 1·1 | 1·0 |
| Carrot | 10·0 | 0·7 | 1·0 |
| Egg—yolk | 0·0 | 15·0 | 33·0 |
| Milk | 4·5 | 3·2 | 3·6 |
| Orange | 20·0 | 1·0 | 1·0 |
| Potato | 12·0 | 1·5 | 0·5 |

As we have said, different people need different amounts of energy, depending on the job they are doing. Today you might have been active and playing games. Now you are quiet. The chart below shows approximately how much energy a person needs, depending on their age, sex and occupation. If a person eats food and therefore stores up energy in excess of bodily needs he or she will almost certainly begin to put on too much weight, though by how much can vary considerably from person to person.

### ENERGY NEEDED EACH DAY

| Individual | Kilojoules needed |
|---|---|
| 3-year-old child (boy or girl) | 4,500 |
| 9-year-old girl | 9,000 |
| 9-year-old boy | 10,000 |
| 15-year-old girl | 13,000 |
| 15-year-old boy | 15,500 |
| Patient in hospital (in bed) | 7,500 |
| Secretary (female) | 10,000 |
| Secretary (male) | 12,000 |
| Bricklayer | 15,000 |
| Labourer on building site | 20,000 |
| Senior citizen | 8,500 |

**fat**

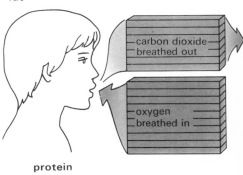

carbon dioxide breathed out

oxygen breathed in

**protein**

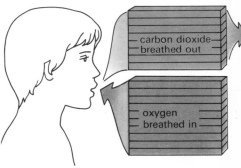

carbon dioxide breathed out

oxygen breathed in

**carbohydrate**

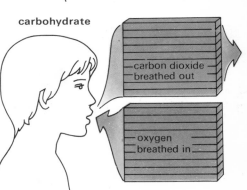

carbon dioxide breathed out

oxygen breathed in

When foods are broken down, oxygen is consumed and carbon dioxide given off is known as the respiratory quotient (RQ). As you will see, it varies with different foods. The amount of oxygen used and carbon dioxide given off during the breakdown of carbohydrates is the same.

27

# Food for our bodies

Fortunately, most of us in this country get enough to eat. But you've probably seen pictures on television and in magazines of people in some parts of the world who do not have enough food. Two out of every three people in the world suffer from the effects of too little food, or at any rate, not enough of the right kinds of food.

To keep healthy we need a balanced diet. Make a list of all the things you eat during a week. You need carbohydrates, fats and proteins, together with small amounts of vitamins (see chart) and some minerals – all this and water as well. Water, whether on its own or in other foodstuffs, is vitally important because about 70 per cent of our body is made up of this liquid.

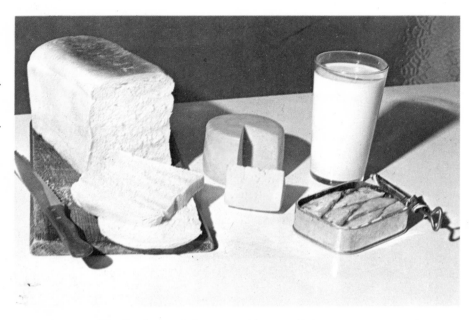

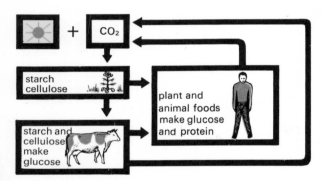

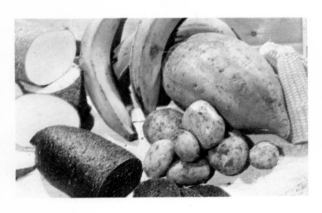

*Above* Foods containing calcium, including cheese, milk, fish and enriched bread, are very important for our health. Calcium is needed by the body to help build strong bones and teeth.

*Left* Carbohydrates are made by plants. They use sunlight, water and carbon dioxide. Only plants with the green pigment chlorophyll can actually make the carbohydrates. Once the plant has made its food, it may be eaten directly by man or by animals, like sheep and cows, which we will then eat as meat.

*Left* The basic foods we eat, including potatoes and bread, contain high levels of carbohydrates. By eating these the body gets its essential supplies.

*Right* If a child lacks vitamin D and calcium in its diet, the bones become soft and bend.

In the X-ray *(far right)* the child has rickets. The light edges on the right joint show where treatment has been carried out. The left-hand X-ray shows normal growth.

Almost all the energy we need comes from carbohydrates and fats, a little also coming from proteins. Minerals are very important in various parts of our body. Bones (page 10) are made mostly of minerals called calcium and potassium and teeth mainly of calcium and phosphate. Our nerves also need minerals to work properly. Iron is important in the blood, and people who do not have enough suffer from anaemia.

Compared with the large quantities of carbohydrates we need, the amount of vitamins required by the body is small, although they are essential to health.

Carbohydrates make up the biggest part of our diet, and most of

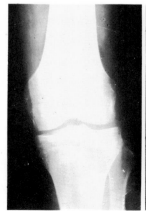

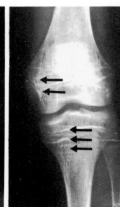

these consist either of starch or are sweet. Potatoes have a lot of starch in them, and pastry and cereal items are also starchy. But bread, made from the flour of wheat or some other cereal crop, is our most important source of carbohydrates. Once the carbohydrates are in our bodies, they will be changed to glucose, which we need for energy.

We need fat to help insulate us. Most of the fats which we eat come from the fat on meat, from eggs, milk, and the other products made from milk, like butter, and from vegetable oils. If we have too much fat in the body, the excess will be stored. Some people use up more fat than others. There are people who can eat a great deal of food and yet stay thin. In times of need the fat can be used to provide energy. People who diet, for example, use up their reserves of stored fats first.

Most of our proteins come from meat, fish, cheese, eggs, milk and beans. All our foods—fats, carbohydrates and proteins—contain carbon, hydrogen, and oxygen, but it is only the proteins which contain nitrogen as well. The body uses proteins when making new cells. Proteins provide the body's building blocks, and even

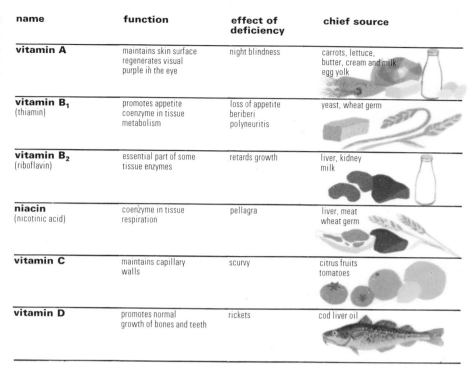

| name | function | effect of deficiency | chief source |
|---|---|---|---|
| vitamin A | maintains skin surface regenerates visual purple in the eye | night blindness | carrots, lettuce, butter, cream and milk egg yolk |
| vitamin B₁ (thiamin) | promotes appetite coenzyme in tissue metabolism | loss of appetite beriberi polyneuritis | yeast, wheat germ |
| vitamin B₂ (riboflavin) | essential part of some tissue enzymes | retards growth | liver, kidney milk |
| niacin (nicotinic acid) | coenzyme in tissue respiration | pellagra | liver, meat wheat germ |
| vitamin C | maintains capillary walls | scurvy | citrus fruits tomatoes |
| vitamin D | promotes normal growth of bones and teeth | rickets | cod liver oil |

though we might have a plentiful supply of carbohydrates and fats, we couldn't live without some proteins.

The body needs twenty different kinds of mineral. Although we know that calcium is important for our teeth and bones and that fluoride helps to prevent our teeth from decaying, we do not know how some of the others work.

If we had a diet which consisted only of carbohydrates, fats and proteins, we would die unless we also had vitamins. Because they occur only in very small amounts, they took a long time to discover. At first four were identified—A, B, C, and D. Now we know that there are many more. The story of how Englishmen became known as Limeys has to do with vitamins. At one time sailors at sea suffered badly from a disease called scurvy which caused blood vessels under the skin to burst and the hair and teeth to fall out. It could easily be fatal. Scurvy was due to a lack of fresh fruit and vegetables, and therefore of vitamin C, in their diet. English sea captains were some of the first to include fresh fruit in their ships' rations, as an antidote to scurvy. The fruit chosen was often limes, hence the nickname.

*Above* The chart shows where our vitamins come from. Although these substances are found only in small amounts, they are essential for a healthy body. When they are lacking, a number of diseases occur. Today our diet is such that it usually contains adequate supplies. Vitamins in food are often destroyed by heating, and so supplements in the form of pills may be taken.

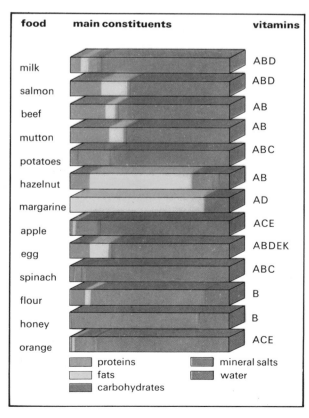

| food | main constituents | vitamins |
|---|---|---|
| milk | | ABD |
| salmon | | ABD |
| beef | | AB |
| mutton | | AB |
| potatoes | | ABC |
| hazelnut | | AB |
| margarine | | AD |
| apple | | ACE |
| egg | | ABDEK |
| spinach | | ABC |
| flour | | B |
| honey | | B |
| orange | | ACE |

proteins    mineral salts
fats    water
carbohydrates

*Left* Some foods, like eggs, are rich in a wide variety of vitamins. Others, like flour, contain only one. We need to have a diet which supplies us with an adequate supply of proteins, fats and carbohydrates, as well as with small quantities of minerals. The diagram compares various food substances and shows how each is made up.

# Teeth

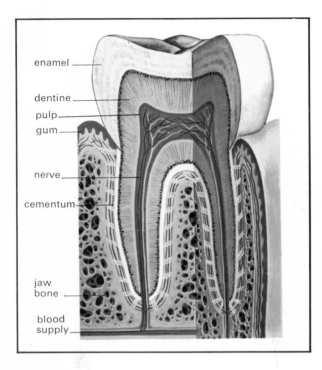

enamel

dentine

pulp

gum

nerve

cementum

jaw bone

blood supply

*Left* Cross-section through a human tooth. Although this illustration is of a molar tooth, all are made up in the same way. The outside of the tooth is covered with hard enamel for protection. Under this is dentine which is much softer. The centre of the tooth has pulp in it, and this is supplied with blood. Nerves also go to each tooth, so that there is some warning if anything goes wrong. You can see that the pointed parts of the tooth, usually called the roots, hold it firmly in the jaw. A child's milk teeth fall out because the second set is underneath. An adult sometimes has to have bad teeth extracted. Because molar teeth are well down in the gums they take a lot of pulling to remove them from the jaw.

The teeth have got to be tough to deal with all the hard work they have to do. Although they are different shapes, they are all made up in the same way. The tooth is alive and has a supply of blood and nerves. You've probably found out about the nerves if you have had toothache! The enamel is a hard outer covering which is very strong and can stand up to great wear and tear. Most of the tooth consists of dentine. The long roots of the tooth hold it firmly in the jaw-bone.

At some time or other most people suffer from toothache, which is usually, but not always, caused by bad teeth. Bacteria are always around, ready to attack when they get the chance. The bacteria feed on pieces of food trapped between the gums and teeth. As they do so they produce acids that gradually dissolve the enamel. Sugary and starchy foods produce the most acid

Have a look at your teeth in a mirror. You will see that they are not all the same. There are four different types. At the front are the incisors, next the canines, then the premolars and lastly the molars.

Because the food we eat is varied, each type of tooth has its own job to do. Get a biscuit and put it to your mouth. What do the incisors do? They bite off a piece which is then pushed by the tongue to the teeth at the back. See if you can keep it at the front and notice how long it takes you to chew it. We don't use all our teeth all of the time. It depends on the sort of food we are eating. The canines which are used for piercing and tearing flesh are not very well developed in humans because we do not need to tear flesh in the same way that, say, a dog does. Premolars and molars are used for grinding the food, making it easier to swallow.

How many teeth do you have? It will depend how old you are. A four-year-old child has only twenty, compared with thirty-two in an adult's mouth. As you grow older, the jaw grows, making room for more teeth.

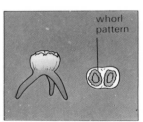

molars   premolars   canines   incisors

*Above* An adult has thirty-two teeth. There are four different sorts: the incisors at the front, with the canines next to these. Towards the back of the mouth are the premolars and molars. Each line shows the teeth in *half* the mouth. There are the same sort of teeth in the top and bottom sets. The premolars and molars in the upper mouth have extra roots to anchor them into the jaw.

*Above* This is a baby's molar tooth, which is very different from the one which will replace it. The roots are spread out, and the surface of the tooth is very uneven.

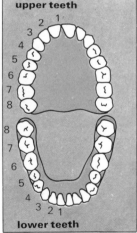

*Above* A view of the teeth as they are arranged in the mouth. You can compare the numbers here with those on the diagram on the left. The back teeth fit on to each other, but the front ones do not. When the teeth come together to grind food, they do it quickly and efficiently.

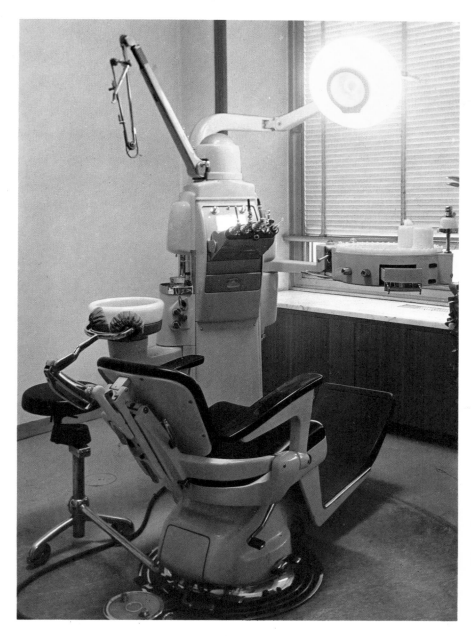

you an injection to numb the nerves, so that you can't feel the pain when he works on the tooth.

When people have several teeth extracted, false ones can be made. A wax impression is taken of a person's mouth, and a plaster cast is made from this. Teeth are made either from porcelain or plastic. Although plastic teeth are easier to make, porcelain ones wear better.

Sometimes teeth grow out of the jaw at the wrong angle, or there are large gaps between them. The dentist will usually place a wire brace round the teeth, and this helps to strengthen them or draw them together. Once corrected, the wire is removed.

Scientists carrying out research have found that fluoride helps to strengthen the enamel on the teeth. It is added to drinking-water in some areas. Brushing teeth with toothpaste containing fluoride also helps. Dentists can treat the teeth with fluoride, and this will have the same effect as having fluoride in the drinking-water. You can protect your teeth if you make sure that you brush them carefully after every meal.

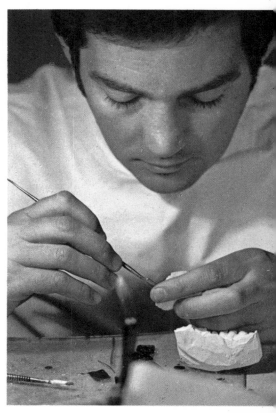

when the bacteria feed on them. Although it may take a while, a hole will be worn through the enamel, and the acids will then reach the dentine. The tooth will now begin to ache, but if decay reaches the pulp it will be extremely painful and infection may spread.

Today a dentist can deal with the decay. He will drill out the rotten part, making sure that all of it is removed. He then fills the cavity with material which will not decay. This is usually made up of silver, with small amounts of zinc and copper, which is then mixed with mercury.

Sometimes a tooth is too far

*Above* A modern dentist's surgery, with all the equipment the dentist will need close at hand.

*Right* A wax cast is made of a person's mouth, and from this a plaster replica will be produced. Here a dental mechanic is making a slight adjustment to the impression. The plastic base plate will be moulded from this, and then the artificial (false) teeth will be put in position. Teeth are usually made from hard plastic, although porcelain is also used.

decayed, and if the dentist drilled away all the bad part, there would not be anything for the filling to be attached to, and so he will extract it. When either filling or taking out a tooth, the dentist will usually give

# Digestion

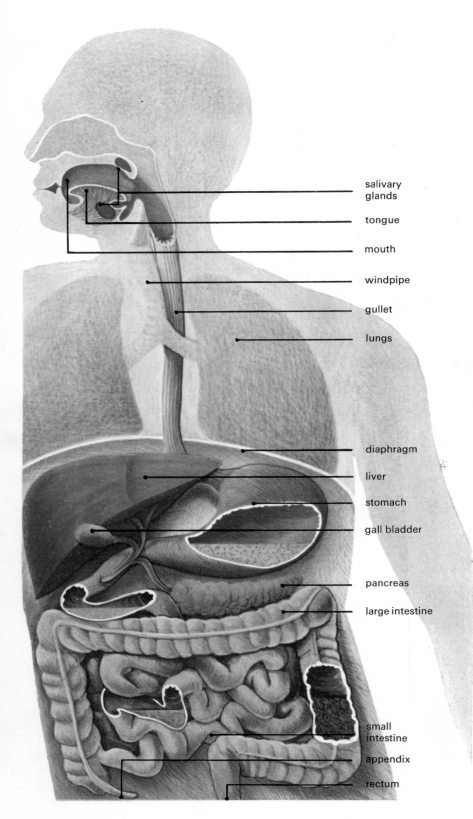

salivary glands

tongue

mouth

windpipe

gullet

lungs

diaphragm

liver

stomach

gall bladder

pancreas

large intestine

small intestine

appendix

rectum

Eat a biscuit or a slice of bread and take note of how you go about it. You bite the food and chew it up into a sort of pulp, softening it at the same time with saliva secreted from glands in your mouth. By the time you are ready to swallow the food it has already undergone a considerable change. But this is only the start of a long and complicated process of digestion once you have swallowed the food and it has proceeded down your gullet, or oesophagus, and into your stomach.

There are a number of stages in the process of digestion. First the food is broken up by the teeth, and the tongue then helps to mix the food with the saliva. In the saliva there is an enzyme called ptyalin, which changes sugar into starch. The salivary glands are continuously secreting saliva into the mouth. Have you noticed how active they are when you smell something good? Your mouth waters! This is a good example of the way one action in the body is linked with another.

Once a mouthful of food is mixed thoroughly, it will be swallowed. If you look at the diagram, you will see how the food gets into the stomach. The wall of the oesophagus is made of muscle so that it can squeeze the food along. The stomach itself is like an elastic bag. It can change shape to make room for all the contents of a meal. This might be quite a large amount and will include all that we drink as well. Although we don't actually feel it, the muscles of the stomach wall are constantly churning the food and mixing it with other chemicals. Another enzyme called

The digestive system starts at the mouth. Food placed here is chewed, mixed with saliva, and then passed down the gullet (oesophagus) into the stomach. Here various substances are added, and the food is thoroughly mixed before it is passed into the small intestine. The useful materials are broken down into simpler substances, which can be used by the body, and are taken away by the blood. The solid, undigested waste, known as faeces, continues along the large intestine to the rectum.

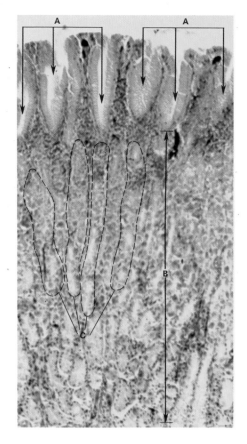

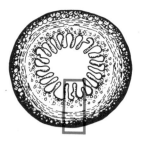

*Left* A magnified section of the stomach wall. The lining is folded (A). The gastric glands (C) are found in tissues marked B. *Above* The small projections, called villi, stick out from the wall of the small intestine so that more food can be absorbed.

*Right* A magnified section of the villi to show their make-up. Blood comes close to the digested food in the intestine, and the food is absorbed through the thin walls of the capillaries. Once in the blood, the food can be taken all over the body and used by the cells.

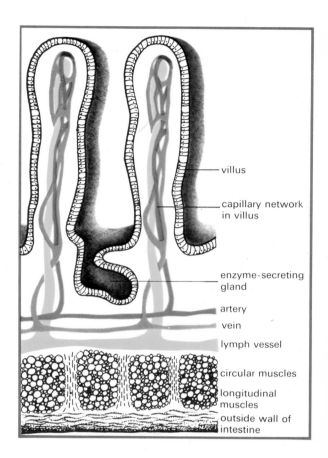

villus

capillary network in villus

enzyme-secreting gland

artery

vein

lymph vessel

circular muscles

longitudinal muscles

outside wall of intestine

pepsin is added and helps to break down the proteins. At the same time, some of the cells in the stomach wall produce hydrochloric acid. This is quite weak, but pepsin will work only if there is acid in the stomach. A coating of mucin prevents the stomach wall from being attacked by the acid. Rennin is another enzyme and this starts to work on milk. Rennin is very important in young children when, for the first weeks of their life, they feed only on milk. With all these things added and with the help of the churning action the stomach changes the food into a porridge-like material called chyme. The time the stomach needs to achieve this will vary according to the type of food it is handling. Bread and pastry are quickly broken up by the stomach's chemical action. Meat takes longer. Fats stay in the stomach for the greatest length of time. You may have heard someone say that a meal 'laid heavy on the stomach'. This usually refers to greasy meals because they remain there longer than others.

The stomach narrows towards the far end, and a ring of muscle, called the pyloric sphincter, controls the exit. When it opens, the stomach squeezes food out into the small intestine. The adjective 'small' only refers to the width of this intestinal tube. In fact it is between six and seven metres (19 and 23 ft) long in an adult. The first part is called the duodenum and close by is an organ called the pancreas. This is very important because it produces the enzymes which are sent into the intestine. At the same time bile from the liver is also added. The food so far has been worked on by the stomach, but it isn't yet ready to be used by the body. Enzymes from the pancreas, as well as those which are made in the wall of the intestine, are added and help with further digestion.

The walls of the small intestine are not smooth, but are covered with a large number of villi, tiny 'fingers' which stick out, increasing the surface area of the intestine for absorption. Each of the villi contains a network of blood capillaries. The walls of the villi are very thin so that the liquid food can pass through them. Amino acids (proteins), glu-

cose, fats and water then travel into the bloodstream.

There is a large part of food which we cannot use. We cannot break down the cellulose in greens. So the waste, together with a good deal of water, has to be disposed of. It goes into the large intestine. This is much wider than the small intestine. The water from the waste will go back into the blood, and what remains is a partly solid waste. To help this move along mucin is added. The waste will eventually reach the rectum, and when there is enough it will be discharged from the body as faeces.

One of the body's most vital organs is the liver. In some respects it is like an incinerator, burning up certain waste or toxic substances. It can also be compared to a filter system and to an energy storehouse. In all it has some five hundred different tasks to do. Because of its importance, it isn't surprising that the liver is the largest organ in our bodies. In an adult is weighs between 1·3 and 1·8 kg (3–4 lb). Once it becomes damaged, the body doesn't work properly, because the

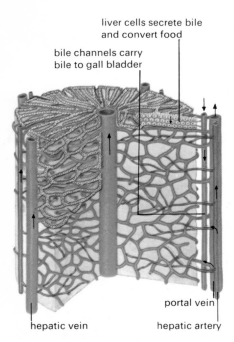

liver cells secrete bile
and convert food

bile channels carry
bile to gall bladder

portal vein

hepatic vein

hepatic artery

*Above* Cross-section of a liver lobule.

*Below* The liver is the largest organ in the body and is divided into four lobes. Oxygen arrives in the hepatic artery and digested food in the portal vein.

liver is responsible for doing so many jobs.

You will see from the diagram where the liver is found in the body. It's in the upper part of the abdomen, a little to the right of, and partly above, the stomach. While we are at rest, about one-quarter of the body's blood – 5 litres (11 US pints) – is in the liver. As activity starts up, the liver quickly sends between 1 and 1½ litres (2–3 US pints) of blood to other organs.

You will remember that the food which we take into the body is made up of carbohydrates, proteins and fats. Since they can't be used as they are, they are broken down during the process of digestion. Now they are in a simpler form which can be carried in the bloodstream and taken to all parts of the body as required. Some of these simpler materials are converted by the liver for storage in the body. The liver also changes other chemicals so that they can be used by the body.

As well as doing this job, the liver can also deal with some poisons called toxins which get into the body from time to time. Although many people take alcohol without its doing them any harm, this is a toxic liquid as far as the body is concerned. The liver will deal with it and make it harmless. When we are ill, it may be necessary for the doctor to give us drugs. If these were allowed to stay in the body, they would soon become dangerous. After they have finished their task, it is the liver which will break them down and make them harmless.

Because they work continuously, the red blood cells wear out after about four months. Instead of being wasted they are broken down in the liver and the spleen, and the iron which is released can be used again to form new cells.

The liver is an unusual shape. There are four parts, called lobes, which can easily be seen. Under the microscope we can see much more. There are many thousands of cells which are built up into columns, called lobules. These are supplied with plenty of blood. Some cells

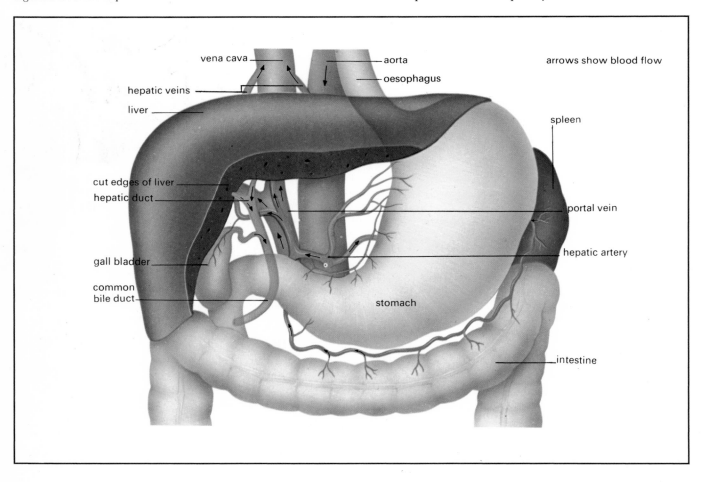

vena cava

aorta

oesophagus

arrows show blood flow

hepatic veins

liver

spleen

cut edges of liver

hepatic duct

portal vein

hepatic artery

gall bladder

common bile duct

stomach

intestine

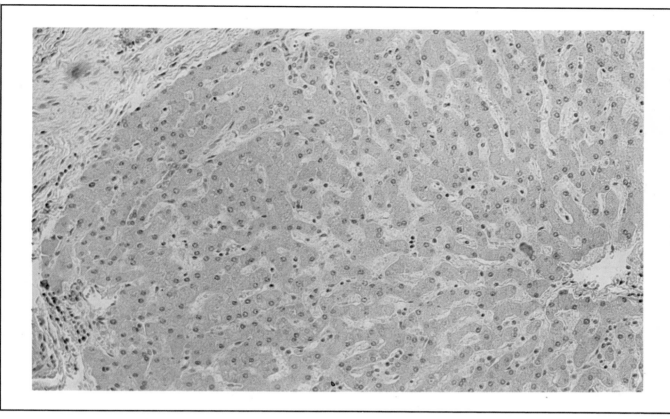

make a liquid called bile, which is poured into ducts and stored in the gall bladder.

As the liver is a very important organ, it is supplied with two lots of blood. Oxygen is needed by the cells in the liver, just as it is by cells in other parts of the body. This blood is brought by the hepatic artery. Blood also comes to it in the portal vein. You will remember that the digested food leaves the small intestine and goes into the blood. Eventually the capillaries join up, and the food is carried in the hepatic portal vein. Having circulated through the liver, the blood has given up its oxygen and food and leaves in the hepatic vein.

Blood passes through spaces between the liver cells and food substances are taken out. They will be changed into storage foods in the liver until they are needed by the body. A very important hormone called insulin helps to change the glucose to glycogen. When the body needs an extra supply of glucose for energy, the glycogen can be changed back into glucose. It can then go back into the blood to be taken to the muscles. Both fats and proteins

*Above* A healthy liver lobule shown in a photomicrograph. The white 'blob' is a blood vessel.

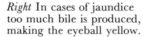

*Right* In cases of jaundice too much bile is produced, making the eyeball yellow.

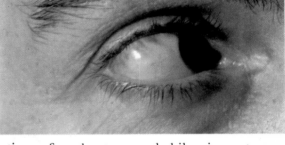

can be stored in the liver. In times of need fat can be broken down so that it can be used for energy. Other by-products of digestion which the body does not need will be chemically broken down by the liver and made into urea. This goes into the blood travelling from the liver to the kidneys, where it will be mixed with water and discharged from the body as urine.

The liver makes nearly a litre of bile every day. It doesn't need it all, and some is stored in the gall bladder. There are some salts in the bile, and these help with the digestion of fats. There are also a lot of waste products in the bile, as well as bile pigments. The latter are left when the blood cells are broken down. When the liver does not work prop-

erly, too much bile pigment may be produced, and then jaundice develops. This makes the skin and the eyeballs yellow.

Diseases of the liver can occur, including hepatitis, when a virus destroys some of the liver cells. People who drink too much alcohol may get cirrhosis, which also kills off some of the cells.

# Getting rid of waste

We have read on page 32 how food is prepared in the mouth and stomach for digestion by the body as it passes through the intestines, and how those solids not absorbed into the bloodstream are expelled as faeces. These faeces are, of course, a form of waste matter, but they are not of the same order of waste as that produced by the body as it converts food into energy. How the body rids itself of this kind of waste is called excretion.

The principal organs of excretion are the kidneys. These are bean shaped, reddish-brown in colour, and situated in the small of the back on either side of the spine. In an adult they are about 11 cm ($4\frac{1}{2}$ in) long and 6 cm ($2\frac{1}{2}$ in) broad.

The kidneys are a type of blood filter. They remove from the blood waste matter and other impurities, and also maintain the correct proportion of water and other substances in the blood. The blood enters them through the renal artery. Inside each kidney the renal artery splits up into a network of over a million capillaries. Each of these forms itself into a kind of twisted knot called a glomerulus, and this is surrounded by a special capsule of very thin, porous tissue. The section of capillary leading into each glomerulus is larger than the section leading away from it, so that blood pressure is built up as it flows through. Under this pressure many substances in the blood pass as a solution through the tissue of the glomerulus and into the capsule. From there the solution passes into a tube, or tubule, which is intertwined with a network of blood vessels leading from the glomerulus. Those substances in the solution which the body needs are then re-absorbed into the blood; the remainder of the solution continues along the tubule to the bladder. This is something like a balloon which swells in size as urine collects in it, until there is enough to be expelled from the body.

Urine is a solution mainly of urea in water. During the digestive process of breaking down food into

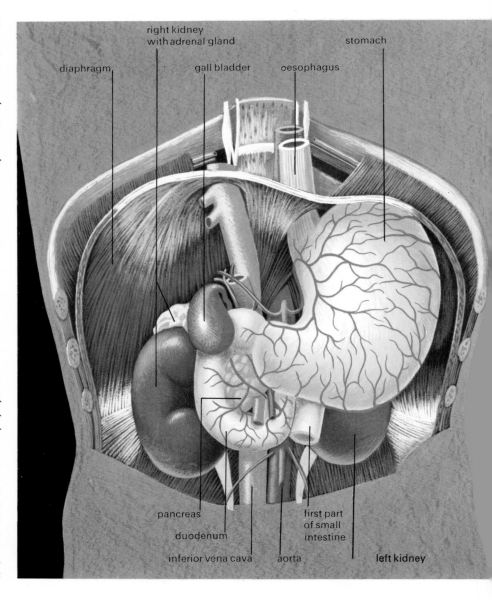

its various constituents and building them up again into substances the body can use as energy, ammonia is produced. This is extremely poisonous and so the liver converts it, with carbon dioxide, into the less harmful chemical urea. It usually forms only about four per cent of the urine, though this proportion can vary depending upon how much water there is in the body at a particular time and how much of this the kidneys retain in the blood.

Until recently, if a person's kidneys stopped working properly they

The digestive organs of the abdomen showing the position of the kidneys behind and a little below the stomach. The kidneys filter and purify the blood and also regulate the many complicated chemical changes which take place during digestion and the conversion of food into energy. Blood passes through them at the rate of about one and a quarter litres ($2\frac{1}{2}$ US pints) every minute.

soon died, because harmful materials quickly accumulated in the blood and poisoned the body. Today there are machines which can perform the kidney's functions. The patient is connected to the

A kidney machine in operation. The patient is connected up to the machine and his entire blood supply is circulated through the machine for cleansing. The size and complexity of the apparatus underlines the marvellous job which our own relatively small and compact kidneys carry out every minute of the day.

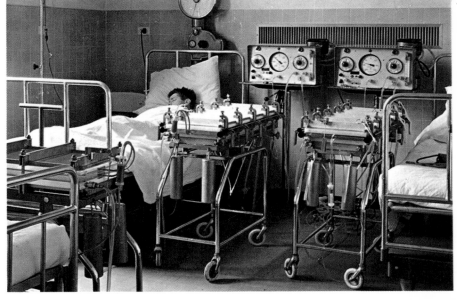

machine while his or her entire blood supply is passed through it. A person with failed kidneys might have to spend two days every week on a kidney machine. Today people with failed or damaged kidneys may also receive a transplant.

Another important way in which the body excretes waste and excess water is through sweating. Beneath the surface of the skin are sweat glands. These are surrounded by tiny blood capillaries. The walls of the capillaries and of the sweat glands allow excess water and impurities to pass from one to the other. Once in the sweat gland, the liquid waste is discharged through pores in the skin. On average we get rid of nearly a litre (2 US pints) of water a day through sweat, though in hot weather, or as a result of strenuous exercise, we might sweat out of our bodies as much as 2 litres (4 US pints) in an hour. In extreme conditions a person can sweat up to as much as 4 litres (8 US pints) in an hour.

Sweating also serves a very valuable purpose in helping to regulate body temperature. The internal organs need to be kept at a fairly constant temperature. The burning up of food as energy during exercise rapidly increases the body's own heat. Sweat on the surface of the skin rapidly evaporates and cools the body down again. In the same way it helps to keep our bodies cool in warm surroundings. There is

a close connection here between sweating and the production of urine. In hot weather or during periods of hard physical exercise, we do not urinate as much as usual because we are excreting more excess water as sweat. At the same time, the sweat glands cannot regulate the balance of chemicals within the blood in the way that the kidneys are able to do. One of the ingredients of sweat is sodium chloride, or common salt. A certain amount of salt is essential to the body, but the sweat glands cannot

control this, and as long as they go on producing sweat so the body will be losing salt. In very hot weather, therefore, people often need more salt in their diet to compensate for that lost through sweat.

The lungs are also organs of excretion, expelling carbon dioxide and more excess water. We breathe this out as vapour, as we can see clearly for ourselves if we watch our breath condense on a relatively cold surface like a window pane. We lose about another half litre (1 US pint) of water a day through the lungs.

The excretory system of the kidneys. The renal artery carries blood to the kidneys where it is purified and then returned to the bloodstream by the renal vein. Waste matter and excess water (urine) proceed down the ureters to the bladder where it is collected and finally expelled from the body.

kidney

renal vein

renal artery

ureter

bladder

# Feeling

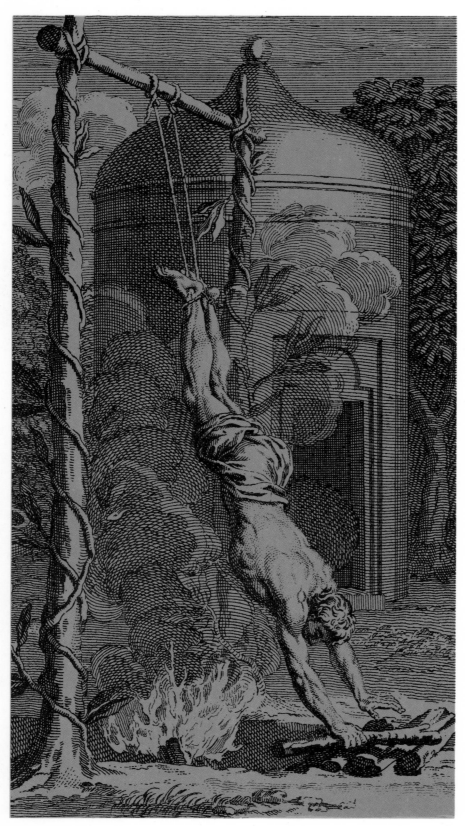

Pinch yourself! If you did it hard enough, it probably hurt, although not quite as much as the last time someone kicked you! You probably exclaimed that it hurt. What you were really saying was that you felt pain. But while we don't usually like pain, it is very important to us. Imagine having no feelings and accidentally putting your hand on a very hot kettle. Think what would happen. You would probably have burnt you whole hand. But if you do touch the kettle, you quickly remove your hand because you feel pain. This is a means of warning the body. There are other pains which tell us that something is wrong: toothache, although very unpleasant, is a warning that all is not well. We can usually take the necessary action when we feel this sort of pain. Although we can't actually measure pain, we do have different ways of describing it. An ache might be a dull pain, whereas a sharp pain, like that when you burn a finger, will hurt more.

Most of our pains don't last very long. Pinch yourself again and see how long the pain lasts. It goes quite quickly. A burn will be painful for much longer, and someone suffering from arthritis will usually be in pain for a long while. Usually, pain affects only parts of our bodies.

How do we feel pain? It's all due to nerves. When your finger touches a hot kettle, the nerve endings in the fingers send tiny electrical signals to the central nervous system (CNS). When the impulses have reached the CNS, they are interpreted, and a signal is sent back to the arm so that we move the limb away and feel pain in the finger almost immediately. There are other impulses going to the CNS, and scientists think that those of pain are no different until they get to the spinal

Some people are able to withstand greater pain than others. This Hindu mystic is about to place his hands in the fire. Scientists think that it is possible to control some kinds of pain by having a particular attitude of mind and without the use of drugs.

38

cord where a special nerve takes them to the brain, and so we perceive pain.

You might have noticed that when you pinch yourself lightly the pain is less than when you pinch yourself hard. The number of signals going to the brain will dictate the strength of the pain which we feel. When there are a large number of signals every second, then this means that the pain is quite strong. Although we usually feel pain where the damage is, this isn't always so. Someone suffering from heart disease may feel pain in the left arm. People who have lost an arm or a leg may sometimes think they feel pain in the missing limb. Nerves still go to stumps and continue sending messages to the brain, which registers signals from the area and interprets them as being painful.

Not everyone feels the same amount of pain. Someone can have an injection without feeling very much, while another person might be in agony! When considering this, scientists often talk about pain

These Chinese pictures show the places where acupuncture can be practised in the body. This method of curing illnesses was known in China 4,700 years ago. When a person practises acupuncture, he places sterilized metal needles into the skin. If placed correctly they will relieve pain and various ailments.

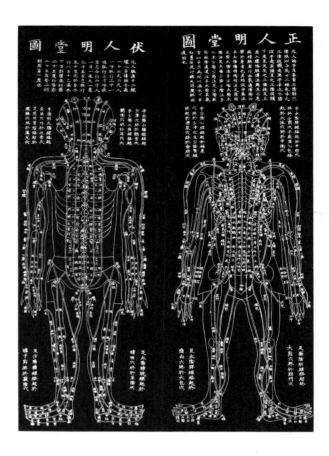

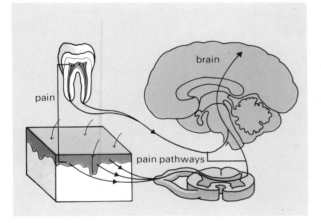

*Left* Different pains in the body travel by different nerve routes.
*Below* Sometimes pain is felt in a different area from its source. In some heart conditions *(left)* pain may be felt in the left arm. A pain in the diaphragm *(right)* may be felt in the neck and shoulders. The nerve impulses from the two regions go into the spinal cord close to each other.

thresholds—the point at which the pain begins. If you press a pin against the skin, you might feel it, whereas a friend might not. A pain threshold in one person is different from that in another. There may be changes in the pain threshold. If you have a severe pain in one part of the body, it might 'disguise' pain which you had in another area.

There are ways of making pain more bearable apart from anaesthetics. If you have a cut leg which hurts and someone is going to bathe it with antiseptic, which might make it hurt even more, you'll probably bite your lip, and this will appear to take the pain away from your leg. You might have heard of acupuncture. People who practise it push pins into the patient's body. No pain is felt. Acupuncture has been used for more than 4,500 years. We cannot be sure how it works, and yet it is often said to be effective when other treatments have failed. There are drugs which can numb the nerves causing the pain. Taking aspirin will usually cure a headache, for example.

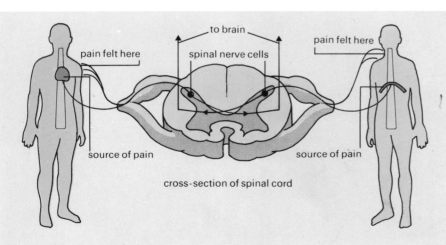

# The ear and hearing

Listen! Did you hear that sound? You probably heard something, because all the time there are noises around us. Some are very loud, others quiet. The noises, caused by vibrations in the air, have reached the ear drum and sent impulses via the inner ear to the brain, which has interpreted them as sounds.

How does the ear receive sound vibrations and transmit them as nerve impulses to the brain? The process starts with the large flap of the outer ear called the pinna. It is the pinna which traps vibrations and directs them down the ear passage to the ear drum, a thin membrane which is stretched tightly across the ear passage. It acts rather like a drum. As vibrations reach this ear drum, they make it vibrate. Immediately behind the ear drum are three small bones called the hammer, anvil and stirrup, because of their shapes. They are the smallest bones to be found in our bodies. The hammer touches the ear drum, so that when this vibrates it will make the hammer move. In turn the hammer is connected to the anvil, which then vibrates. Touching the anvil is the stirrup, which also receives the vibrations.

There is a second drum behind the three bones called the oval window. The stirrup fits into this, and so the oval window picks up the vibrations. The sound waves have now reached the inner ear, but since

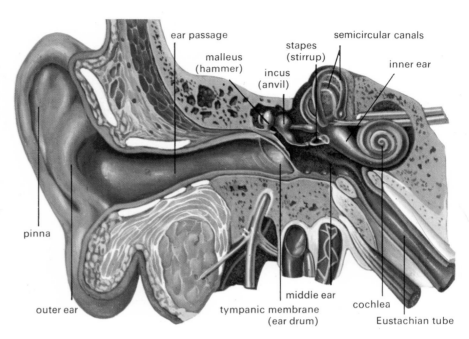

they are still vibrations and we want to hear them as sounds, they have to be changed. The vibrations pass to the long coiled tube called the cochlea. The word comes from the Latin and really means a snail shell. Indeed, the cochlea looks rather like a snail's shell. It is a very complicated organ in the body.

The cochlea has fluid in it, and there are also hair cells with nerves. As the vibrations go through the liquid, they make it move. These movements are picked up by the hairs, and signals are sent along the nerve fibres. These join together to

*Above* The section through a human ear shows how it is made up.
*Below* How sound is translated by the brain. The vibrations travel along the ear channel and reach the ear drum: this vibrates. The hammer picks up the vibrations and passes them to the anvil. The anvil is connected to the stirrup, which picks up the sound waves, and these reach the oval window. This is at the end of the liquid-filled cochlea. As the vibrations go through the liquid, they make it move. The organ of Corti picks up the movements and turns them into signals so that they can be sent to the brain.

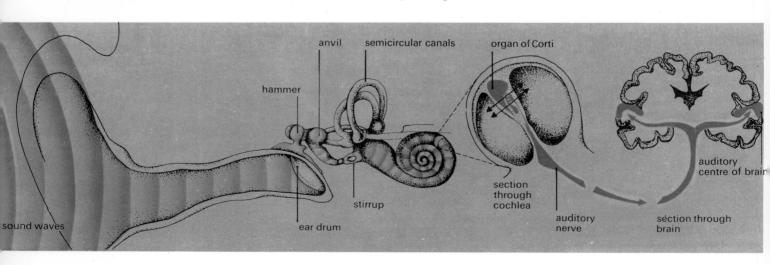

form the auditory nerve, which takes the signals to the brain. It is the brain which will interpret the signals as the sounds we hear. So it is the brain, and not really the ear, which hears.

There is an amazing variety of sounds. If you listen in a crowded place, you will hear the sound of people talking and walking, perhaps even shouting. All the sounds are different. Some are high-pitched; others low-pitched. In the cochlea some of the hairs respond to certain sounds, some to others. We don't hear *all* the sounds around us. Some animals, like dogs, have a greater range of hearing than our own. If we are to hear the sound, it has to vibrate the ear drum. There are also different ranges of sensitivity within the organ of Corti, and this is another reason why we don't hear every sound.

We have said that sounds are caused by vibrations which travel through the air. They also travel through water and solid objects like wood. You can try this. Place a clock on one end of a table. Lay one ear on the table. Can you hear the sound? You should be able to, as it travels through the wood.

Sound waves also travel along land lines, and you can demonstrate this if you make yourself a simple telephone with some cans and string. You will need two cans. Get someone to cut the tops off, so that there are no sharp edges. You will also need a hole drilled in the centre of the bottom of each tin. Now thread some string through the holes, knotting it so that it doesn't fall out. You should now have two tins joined by string. You will need to ask a friend to help now. Talk into one tin can while your friend places the other can over his ear. Can he hear anything? He should be able to, but it may be that the string is too long. You could try to find out how far away your telephone will work by either shortening or lengthening the string. Use a piece of string without knots in it. When you talk into the can, the sounds which you make cause the string to vibrate, and the vibrations will travel along the string.

Sometimes sounds are so loud that they can damage the ear drum.

There are two muscles in the middle ear. One of these is joined to the stirrup, and the other to the ear drum. These are part of a safety system. If a noise is particularly loud, the muscles become shorter—they contract. This makes both the ear drum and the oval window tighter and so stops them from moving backwards and forwards too violently.

The ear isn't concerned only with hearing. It is also important because it helps us to keep our balance. If you swing yourself round and round quite quickly, in the same direction, you will soon lose your balance. How does this happen? The organs of balance are found in the inner ear. There are three semicircular canals in each ear, filled with fluid. These canals are at different angles. In each there are nerves. When the head is moved about, the liquid in the canals also moves. If the movement is sudden, the liquid pushes the nerve cells. These pass impulses to nerve fibres, which in turn are connected to the brain. The brain interprets the impulses and calculates the position and movement of the head. Although the ear is concerned with balance, there are other parts of the body which also contribute to this. Nerve endings in the eyes, the feet, as well as those in muscles and joints, all send their messages to the brain so that the body can keep its balance.

On a boat in rough seas the liquid in your semicircular canals moves about continuously. Although you are still, the brain thinks you are moving and sends out impulses to the body to compensate. But because the body isn't actually moving there is nothing to correct. You may feel sick or dizzy, although the body will usually soon adjust.

There is also a tube, the Eustachian tube, which joins the middle ear to the back of the throat. When you cough or swallow, the tube opens so that the air pressure on either side of the ear drum becomes equal. This helps to prevent damage to the delicate parts of the ear. You have probably felt your ears go 'pop' when going through a tunnel on a train or ascending quickly in a lift. This makes the pressure inside the ear equal to that on the outside.

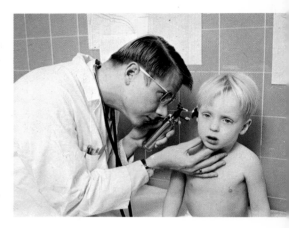

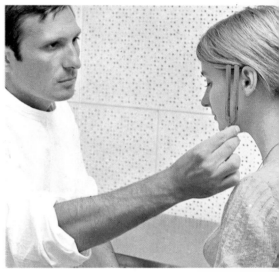

*Above (Top)* Using a special instrument the doctor is able to see inside a child's ear. By careful examination he is able to see whether there is any damage to those parts of the ear which lead from the pinna to the ear drum. By carrying out these and other tests the doctor can find out whether a child is deaf and then suggest ways of dealing with the problem if he is. *(Bottom)* By placing a tuning fork in front of the ear, as well as on the bone behind the ear, the doctor can find out what kind of deafness a person is affected by.

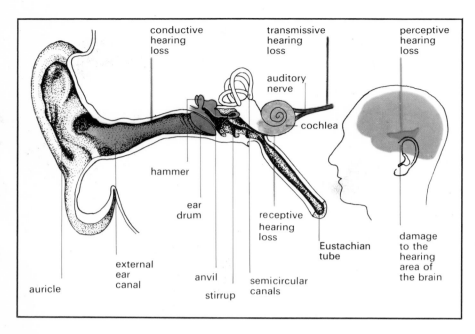

Labels on the upper diagram:
conductive hearing loss · transmissive hearing loss · perceptive hearing loss · auditory nerve · cochlea · hammer · ear drum · receptive hearing loss · Eustachian tube · damage to the hearing area of the brain · external ear canal · anvil · semicircular canals · auricle · stirrup

You are probably lucky and hear quite well. It may sometimes seem a bit of a nuisance, especially when you want to listen to the radio and someone else wants to talk. But try to imagine a world without sounds; no music, no talking, no birds singing. It is difficult for those of us with normal hearing to imagine, but there are people who live in a world of total silence. Even those of us with normal hearing may have this sense seriously damaged by repeated exposure to very loud noise. The volume of sound in some discothèques is known to damage a person's hearing after a period of time. Many factories are also noisy places and those who work in them can become almost stone deaf in course of time.

You can see from the diagram that if various parts of the ear are damaged different types of hearing loss will occur. People may suffer from partial deafness and not be able to hear such things as bird song, or only be able to hear what you say if you shout. Other people suffer from distorted hearing. Although they can hear sounds well enough, these are rather muddled; also, they may not hear everything. If you have ever played a tape backwards or listened to the sound track on a film being run the wrong way, you will have some idea what this means. A person hears the sounds but is not able to make normal sense out of them. When someone suffers from distorted hearing, it is because the nerves have been damaged.

If the ear canal, ear drum or middle ear are damaged, then the sounds which the ear picks up will be fainter. Where the nerves are dam-

aged, either in the inner ear or in that part of our brain which deals with hearing, it usually means that sounds are not clear.

What is called *conductive* hearing loss occurs in the area between the opening of the ear and the three bones on the other side of the ear drum. Some part of the system will be damaged. It might be the ear passage, the drum or one or more of the bones. If the vibrations are not strong enough when they reach the stirrup, this will pass on only weak vibrations to the liquid. When the brain interprets the impulses, they will be heard only as very faint sounds. The person will be 'hard of hearing' and, although not deaf, will certainly find it difficult to hear well.

Inside the inner ear is the organ of Corti. This is very important, because it has got to change the sound waves and make them into tiny electrical impulses so that they can travel along the nerves to the brain. If this very important organ is damaged, people suffer from *receptive* hearing loss. They can usually hear only notes of a certain frequency, depending on the area of damage in the organ of Corti.

When electrical impulses leave the organ of Corti, they will go along the auditory nerve to the cortex of the brain. If the auditory nerves – there is one for each ear – are damaged, they will not carry the impulses. We call hearing loss in this area *transmissive* hearing loss. If the brain is damaged, *perceptive* hearing loss occurs. When either the nerves or the brain are damaged, the sounds will usually be distorted.

Small organisms, known as viruses, may attack the auditory

*Above* Loss of hearing can usually be traced to one or other of two basic causes. If there is damage to the outer or middle ear, then conductive hearing loss occurs, this being the part of the ear which conducts the sound. Damage to either the inner ear or the nervous tissue causes perceptive hearing loss. The person cannot understand – perceive – the sounds, which are difficult to hear. Depending on which part of the ear is damaged, perceptive hearing loss is divided into receptive (receiving), transmissive (transmitting) or strict perceptive deafness.
*Right* The organ of Corti, which is in the cochlea. Vibrations in the cochlea make waves in the liquid, which in turn cause hairs to vibrate. Electrical impulses are interpreted by the brain.

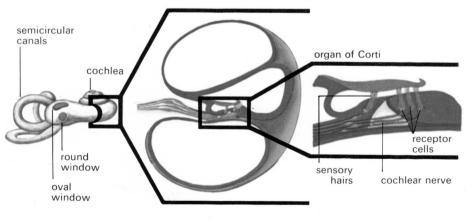

Labels on the lower diagram:
semicircular canals · cochlea · organ of Corti · round window · oval window · sensory hairs · cochlear nerve · receptor cells

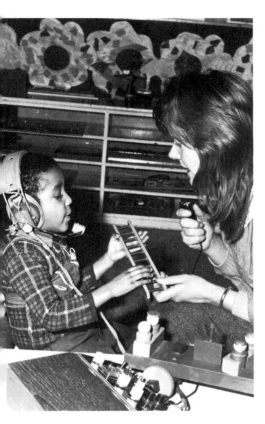

*Above* Deaf children can now be helped to understand sounds with the use of special equipment. By amplifying sounds–making them louder–they can often be distinguished by the brain. Teaching deaf children demands a great deal of patience and understanding between the teacher and the child.
*Below right* Although partially deaf children may be taught in normal classes, those with severe hearing defects are dealt with in special schools. New methods and equipment help specially trained teachers to deal with the deaf child's problems.

nerves, or the cortex, so that hearing is affected. Sometimes not enough oxygen gets to the brain or nerves, and this may cause damage.

While a baby is developing inside the womb, a virus in the mother's blood may go through the umbilical cord (page 65) and pass into the child's blood. When this happens, it can damage the hearing cells growing in the embryo. If the mother catches German measles while pregnant, it is possible that the delicate hearing system of the developing baby will be damaged. If a birth is difficult and the baby suffers temporarily from lack of oxygen damage to hearing can also result.

Alexander Graham Bell made the first electrical hearing aid. Before he developed this, people used to cup hands, or use hollow horns or ear trumpets to increase the sound. Try whispering about half a metre from a friend. See how well they can hear what you are saying. Now make a trumpet from a cone of paper and whisper into this. Is that any better?

In recent years it has been possible to help children who are born deaf. You learnt to speak because you could hear other people talking, and then imitated the sounds you heard. When a child is born deaf, it doesn't hear these sounds and so it cannot learn to talk. Nowadays hearing aids help, and specially trained teachers, using new kinds of equipment, can help the deaf child to communicate properly.

Today doctors and scientists know much more about the way loud noises can affect our hearing as we get older. If the noise level is kept down in factories and at airports, this can help prevent problems later. If girls are immunized against German measles, this helps to lower the number of children who will be born with hearing defects, which the viruses of this disease might cause.

Some young children suffer from ear infections when they have colds. However, these can usually be treated with antibiotics.

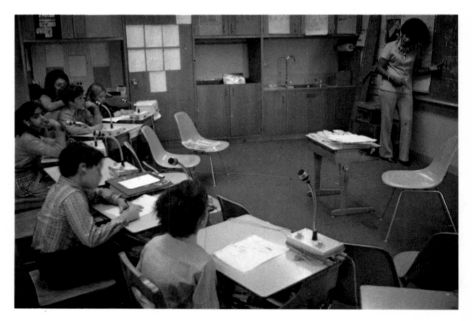

# The eye, sight and blindness

You are probably reading the words in this book and looking at the pictures without any difficulty. But have you ever wondered how it is that we see things?

We see a tree because light falls on it. It might be natural light from the sun's rays or artificial light. On a dark night we wouldn't be able to see the tree, because there is no light. We see objects only when it's light.

It really isn't the eye which sees but the brain. The eye collects the messages in the form of light rays but it has to send these to the brain to be interpreted. There are some light rays, especially ultra-violet ones, which the nerve cells cannot detect.

If you look at the diagram below, you will see that the eye is almost round, and referring back to the skeleton on page 10, you will see that the eyes fit into sockets in the head.

Have a mirror nearby, if possible, while you are reading this. Look into the mirror and notice the whites of your eyes. This is the outer layer. At the front of the eye this layer, called the cornea, is transparent, and light rays can pass through it. Behind the cornea you can see the coloured part of your eye, the iris. In the middle of this is a hole called the pupil. Muscles cause the pupil to dilate—to get bigger—or to constrict—get smaller. In very bright sunlight or in a room with a strong light the rays could damage the eye. In darker conditions we wouldn't be able to see very well. When the muscles alter the size of the pupil, they make the hole larger or smaller so that more or less light can go in.

Behind the iris the lens directs light rays towards the back of the eye. Between the cornea and the

pupil and lens is a watery substance called the aqueous humour, and behind the lens is the jelly-like vitreous humour. Both of these also help to transmit light in the eye.

The cornea could get damaged by specks of dust in the air and so it is covered with a protective film, called the conjunctiva. This does get infected sometimes, and people suffer from conjunctivitis. Although the only time you are likely to see tears is when you cry, the liquid which makes them is always washing the front of the eye to get rid of dust and dirt. The eyelids and the eyelashes also help to stop small objects from actually falling on to the surface of the eye. When you blink you pull the fluid over the eye surface.

If you are looking at this page and you want to look at something to the left or right, you need not necessarily

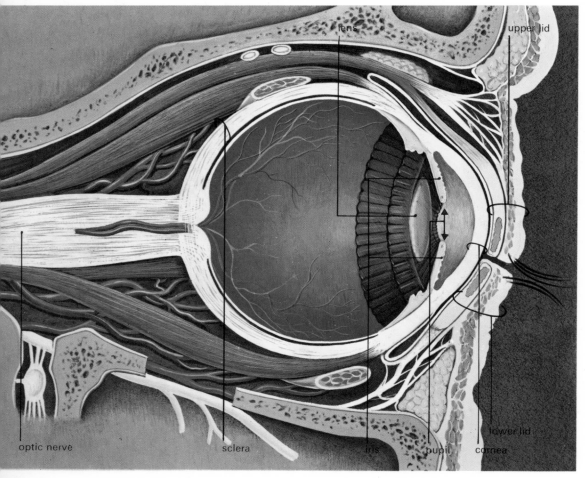

optic nerve · sclera · iris · pupil · cornea · lens · upper lid · lower lid

If we could cut a section through a human eye, this is what we would see. The bony socket protects the delicate parts of the eye. You will see that most of it is enclosed in this protective shell. Various muscles are attached to the eye, and these help us do a number of things. We can move our eye from side to side or up and down without always moving our head. The muscles attached to the lens help this to change shape so that we can focus our eyes on objects which are different distances away.

When light rays have reached the retina, they need to be transmitted to the brain to be interpreted as images. The large optic nerve—one goes from each eye—performs this function.

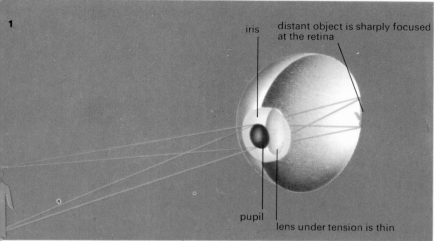

**1**

iris

distant object is sharply focused at the retina

pupil

lens under tension is thin

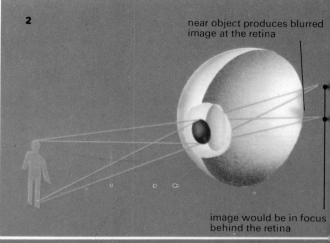

**2**

near object produces blurred image at the retina

image would be in focus behind the retina

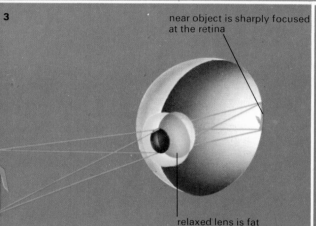

**3**

near object is sharply focused at the retina

relaxed lens is fat

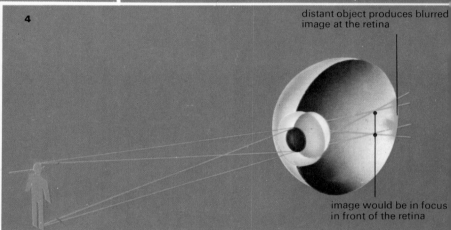

**4**

distant object produces blurred image at the retina

image would be in focus in front of the retina

move your head. The muscles in your eye attached to the eyeball will move it about.

Let's look at how we actually see things. Light, which bounces off objects like the tree, will pass through the cornea. This has a slightly curved surface and it will begin to bend the light rays. The light will then pass through the iris. The muscles will adjust the size of the pupil, depending on how strong the light is. Having gone through the pupil, the light rays now come to the lens. The actual shape of the lens is very important, and muscles attached to it can adjust this shape according to the distance an object may be from the eye. You might be looking at a distant object and then want to look at the words on this page. The muscles will quickly change the shape of the lens, as shown in figures 1 and 3, to ensure that the light rays remain focused on the retina at the back of the eye.

If the lens doesn't change shape when looking at objects at different

*Above* Figure 1 shows that if the lens is in its correct position when looking at a distant object there will be a sharp image on the retina. If it isn't, then we have a blurred image (figure 2). The shape of the lens has to change (figure 3) so that we can focus on a near object. If it doesn't, then again we have a blurred image (figure 4).

*Right* If the eye's own lens does not work properly we need spectacle lenses or contact lenses to achieve correct vision.

distances, then the images become blurred as in figures 2 and 4. To make sure that people can see properly opticians supply glass lenses or contact lenses to do the job of focusing light rays which the eye's own lens is failing to do.

The various parts of the eye, together with any extra lenses which may be necessary, will have focused the light so that it reaches the back of the eye and falls on the area called the retina. Because of the shape of the lens – it is convex (bent outwards on both sides) – the image which reaches the retina is upside down and back to front.

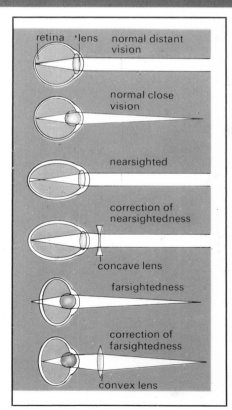

retina  lens  normal distant vision

normal close vision

nearsighted

correction of nearsightedness

concave lens

farsightedness

correction of farsightedness

convex lens

Light has now reached the retina, which is made up of large numbers of two types of cells, rods and cones. These cells, sensitive to light, have been named from their shapes. The rods are more sensitive than the cones but they register only black and white. The rods are spread more evenly over the surface of the retina than the cones. The cones help us to see colours other than black and white. They can work properly only when there is enough light. If there isn't much light, then we see everything as a greyish colour. It's rather like taking a photograph in dull conditions: the print doesn't come out very well. Scientists have found that there are three sorts of cone cells. Some are sensitive to green, some to red and some to blue.

Not surprisingly, perhaps, most of the light entering the eye is likely to fall on the centre of the retina. This part, called the yellow spot, has only cones. When the light is bright, we will see very well, but it is rather a disadvantage in the dark to have only colour-sensitive cone cells in the central part of the retina.

Nerves from the rods and cones join together to form the optic nerve. This will send impulses to the brain to be interpreted as shapes and colours. The brain will process the images in other ways also. Because we have two eyes, two slightly different images are being received at the same time. The brain creates one composite image from these two and thus allows us to see things in depth, that is in three dimensional form, and so to judge distances. The brain also turns the images received on the retina so that they appear the right way up.

Close your eyes and try walking round your own room, somewhere you know very well. The chances are that you will soon start bumping into things and become quite disorientated. That's what would happen if you suddenly went blind, though people who are blind from birth develop their other senses to a far greater degree and are therefore not as helpless as you would be if suddenly deprived of your sight.

Colour blindness is a very real problem for lots of people. Sometimes one of the sets of colour-sensitive cones is missing; sometimes it is more than one. Most people who suffer from colour blindness cannot tell red from green.

To find out whether people suffer from colour blindness the Ishihara

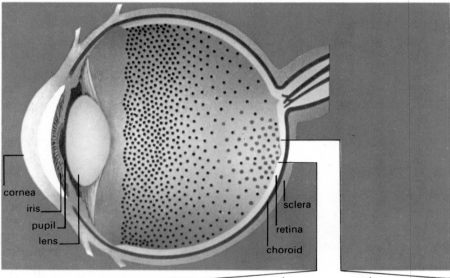

cornea
iris
pupil
lens
sclera
retina
choroid

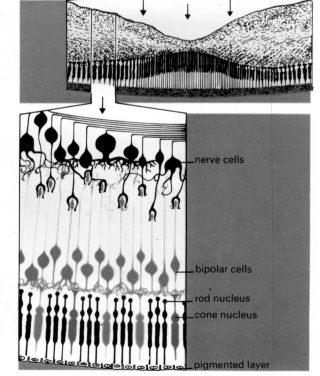

nerve cells

bipolar cells

rod nucleus

cone nucleus

pigmented layer

*Above* Rods and cones are the cells which detect light coming into the eye. The rods are the black dots; the cones are coloured. You can see how they are distributed in the eye.
*Right (Top)* A magnified section of the retina, the light sensitive layer.
*(Bottom)* The retina, magnified again, to show the individual cells. The rods and cones pick up the light rays, and these are passed to the nerve cells, which eventually unite to form the optic nerve. This carries the impulses to the brain.
*Left* Blind people can do most of the things of which sighted people are capable. Here a blind yachtsman coils a halyard. He uses braille maps and can navigate his boat with the use of an audible radio signal. To find his direction he will feel his compass instead of looking at it.

colour cards have been developed. Some of them are shown on this page. Each of the colour cards is covered with a series of dots which, as you can see, are of different colours and sizes. Figures and letters are shown in different-coloured dots. Someone who suffers from colour blindness does not see the letters or numbers. Test yourself to see whether you are affected.

Most people have something wrong with their eyes at least once during their lives. If you don't have anything wrong with yours now, the chances are that you will when you get older. The lenses tend to harden up and so will not change shape. This is when you will need spectacles.

Colours as seen by three people. In 1 the person has normal vision. In 2 there is colour blindness to red. In 3 the person is colour blind to green and is unable to distinguish red from yellow.

1    2    3

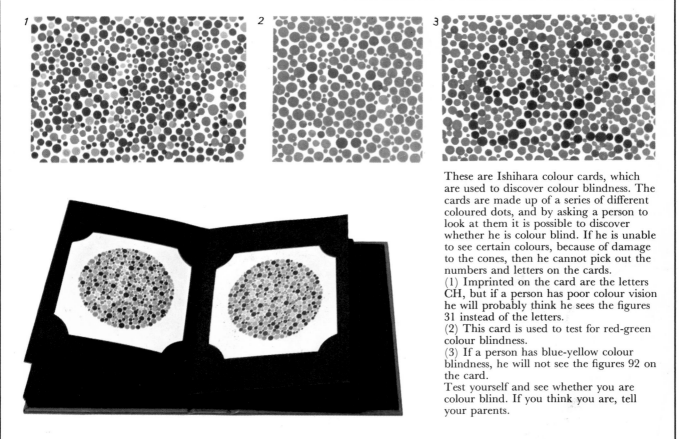

1    2    3

These are Ishihara colour cards, which are used to discover colour blindness. The cards are made up of a series of different coloured dots, and by asking a person to look at them it is possible to discover whether he is colour blind. If he is unable to see certain colours, because of damage to the cones, then he cannot pick out the numbers and letters on the cards.
(1) Imprinted on the card are the letters CH, but if a person has poor colour vision he will probably think he sees the figures 31 instead of the letters.
(2) This card is used to test for red-green colour blindness.
(3) If a person has blue-yellow colour blindness, he will not see the figures 92 on the card.
Test yourself and see whether you are colour blind. If you think you are, tell your parents.

# Taste and smell

Blindfold yourself and then ask someone to put something edible in your mouth. Can you tell what it is? You will probably know what it is by how it feels – your tongue tells you as it moves it about the mouth. But as well as the feel you will also know what it tastes like. Actually, your nose and sense of smell work in close conjunction with your tongue and sense of taste.

How does the tongue detect taste? Over its surface there are a lot of taste buds, as you will see from the drawing. They are one of our five senses and like the others are very important because they tell us something about our surroundings. Although we need a sense of taste so that we can enjoy our food, perhaps the taste buds were more important to our ancestors. When they lived off the land, they soon discovered that bitter things were often, although not always, poisonous. If they picked a wild berry which they didn't know, placed it in their mouths and it tasted bitter, they would have discarded it.

So our taste buds tell us something about the food which we are eating.

You will see in the diagram that different parts of the tongue taste different things. Because the food we eat goes all over the tongue, then some of the taste buds will quickly tell us what kind of thing it is we are eating. In fact, all the things we taste can be divided into four groups. There are those which taste bitter, those which are sour (or acid), those which are sweet, and those which are salty.

The shape of the taste buds is not unlike the shape of buds on a tree, although much smaller. If you look in a mirror and put your tongue out, you will see them as raised pimples on the surface. We have about 9,000 of these in our mouths. Although we usually think of them as being on the tongue – and most are on the upper surface – we also have them on the palate (the roof of the mouth) and in the back of the throat. You will probably have noticed that you can't seem to taste things when you have a cold. This isn't strictly the case. Because taste and smell are closely linked and often work together, when we have a cold it is the smell from a particular food which is masked because our smell cells have been affected.

You will see that there is a small hollow or pocket on the taste bud. As the chemical from the food falls into this scientists think (but are not sure) that it makes the tiny hairs in the hollow react. There are sensory cells inside the taste bud, and these have tiny nerve fibres or fibrils coming from them. Once the sensory cells have collected the information, they will pass it to the nerve fibrils, which in turn will send a signal to the central nervous system. Here it will be interpreted for us, and we will taste whatever is on our tongue.

Of course, the mouth has other nerves too. As well as tasting something 'hot' like curry you also get a burning feeling. This is because other nerve endings have been stimulated.

Although we have only four different types of taste bud, we seem able to distinguish many more smells. It has been estimated that a well-trained person who tests perfumes will be able to distinguish about 10,000 different smells! Just as we remember faces, the brain is

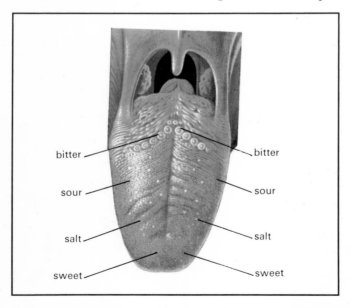

There are four different types of taste bud on the tongue. They help us to distinguish between salty, sour, bitter and sweet things. We taste sweet things at the front and salty things behind. Sour taste buds are behind these, with those for bitter tastes at the back.

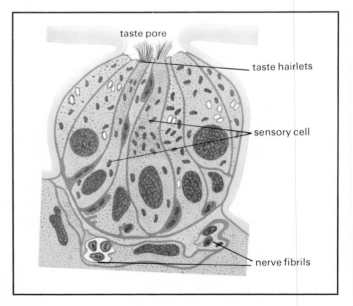

At the top of each taste bud there is a taste pore. When food is put into the mouth, it mixes with the saliva, some of which goes into the taste pore. When it reaches the sensory cell, the dissolved material stimulates it. Nerve fibrils pick up the taste: these join to take messages to the brain.

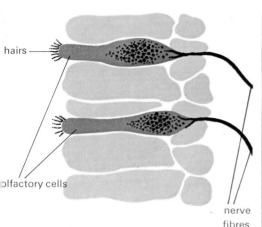

*Above* The olfactory cells which help us to smell things are in the nose. These have to be stimulated if we are to know what each smell is. The nerve fibres take the messages to the brain.

*Right* Because air goes into the body through the nose, this is where the olfactory cells are situated. As the air enters the nose, some of it will reach the cells and stimulate them. The nerve fibres will eventually join together to take these messages to the olfactory lobe which is situated in the brain. If our olfactory cells continue to receive strong smells, we will get used to them. Some smells, like gas and smoke, could be danger signals, and we will take the necessary precautions.

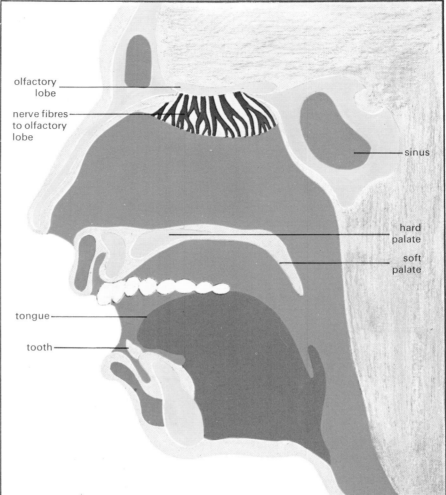

very good at remembering smells, so that once we have smelt something we can usually recall what it is at a later date. After we have had the experience of sniffing burning rubber, next time we smell it we will know what it is. Try to describe a smell to someone else. You will find it almost impossible!

The smell senses, properly called olfactory cells, are found in the upper part of the nose. Although our sense of smell is very good, these cells are removed from the main intake of air: they are really in a blind alley. They are also very small. As soon as a smell reaches them, the owner of the nose will often start to sniff. This helps to get more of the smell to the cells. There are times when the smell is unpleasant, and even though we might stop sniffing, it continues to keep the cells stimulated. As on the taste buds, there are hairs, properly called cilia, on the olfactory cells.

They are not free to wave about in the nose because they are covered with a layer of mucus. The sense of smell is one of the mysteries of the body. We know that we have this sense, but how it actually works has not yet been fully discovered. However, scientists do know that for the smell to be detected it has to 'dissolve' in the mucus. Once the cilia have picked up the smell, the impulses are sent to the brain so that we actually smell something. This happens very quickly, within less than a second after the smell first reached the olfactory cells.

Although we think that we can smell a lot of different things, our sense of smell is not as good as that of a dog. This probably has something to do with the position of the olfactory cells. While ours are hidden away, those of the dog are in the way of the air as it enters and so the air passes over them. There is some-

thing else which helps the dog. The part of the brain dealing with smell is much better developed than in humans!

The sense of smell which often gives us a great deal of pleasure, when we smell fresh spring flowers or new-mown hay, is also very important because it can act as a warning system. If our olfactory cells detect smoke at night, then this might be a warning sign, just as the smell from a leaking gas pipe tells us that something is amiss.

# The nervous system

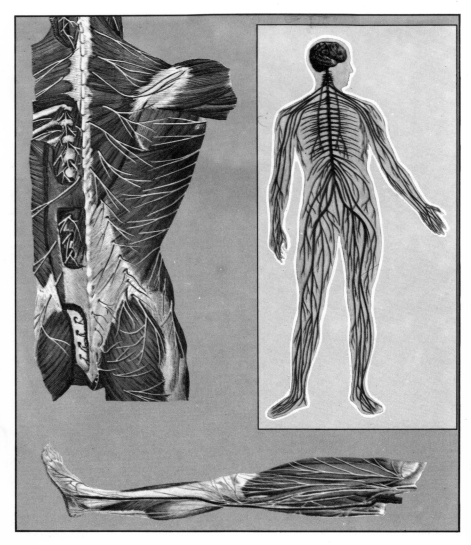

*Left* The human nervous system consists of a vast network of nerve fibres which reach every part of the body. The diagram shows the nerves of the back *(left)*, the whole body *(right)*, and the leg *(below left)*.

*Below* The cell bodies in the brain show up in this photomicrograph as dark patches. The brain has very large numbers of these triangular-shaped cells.

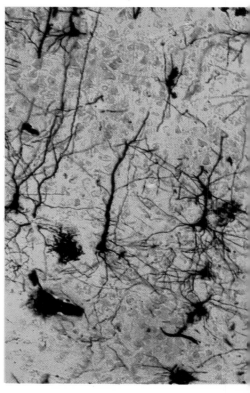

The nervous system is the whole system of nerves by which the brain communicates with the rest of the body and controls and co-ordinates its functions. It is roughly comparable to the telephone lines leading into and out of a central exchange, with thousands of incoming and outgoing calls being processed every second of the day.

The nervous system is, in fact, made up of two quite clearly defined parts. There is the central nervous system (CNS) which consists of the brain and spinal column; and there is the so-called peripheral nervous system, consisting of the nerves which transmit messages to the brain from the senses of sight, hearing, taste, touch and smell and transmit instructions from the brain to the muscles and glands.

Like the rest of our bodies, the nerves are made up of cells. Because of the job they have to do, they are very special cells called neurons. Attached to each neuron is a tail called an axon. Some axons are connected to various cells, like the muscles, which make them contract and relax. Other axons are connected with other nerve cells so that impulses can be passed on. At the end of each neuron there are a lot of small 'wires' sticking out from it. These are dendrites and they receive the messages. A message which passes along the nerve is a very weak electrical current.

Eyes, ears and the other sense organs are part of the nervous system, and as they receive information from our surroundings to pass on to the brain, they are called receptors. It might then be necessary for muscles to react to information received about our surroundings. For example, if you touch something

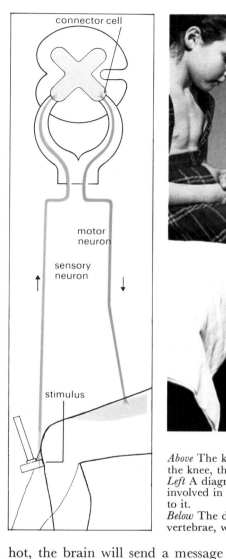

connector cell

motor neuron

sensory neuron

stimulus

will change to the correct size, and so on, all without conscious thought on our part.

When a doctor is giving you a medical examination, he may test your reflex actions to see that the nerves are working properly. Ask a friend to help with this. Get him to sit with his legs crossed so that one leg hangs loosely over the other. Now tap him gently below the knee with the edge of your hand – the little finger edge. The leg should react by jerking upwards. This is called a reflex action. When you hit the leg, you actually touched a tendon which had nerve endings. This sent a message to the spinal cord in the vertebral column. Here it passed via an intermediate neuron, to a motor nerve, which passed it along its axon to make the muscles contract so that the leg jerked. All this happened in less than $\frac{1}{50}$th of a second.

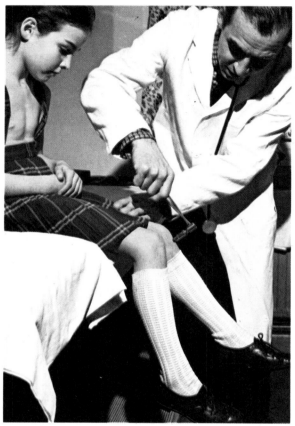

*Above* The knee jerk reflex. When the leg is tapped below the knee, the lower leg will jerk upwards.
*Left* A diagram to show that in this reflex the brain is not involved in the response, although a message will be sent to it.
*Below* The delicate spinal cord inside the individual vertebrae, which make up the spinal column.

hot, the brain will send a message back to the relevant muscles to move your hand away. These are known as the effectors, because they effect (bring about) an action. Nerves which link the receptors to the central nervous system are called sensory nerves – they are involved with the senses. Nerves which link the central nervous system with the effectors are the motor nerves. Different parts of the central nervous system have to be linked together, and there is also a type of nerve which does this.

Many nerves are concerned with the external sense organs, but inside our body activities are going on all the time. Because the nerves which control the inner working of the body do so automatically, they make up what is called the autonomic nervous system. This system makes sure that the kidneys, lungs, bladder, heart, blood vessels, gut,

and the other internal organs, continue to function automatically. It will ensure that the heart beats at the correct rate, that the pupil of the eye

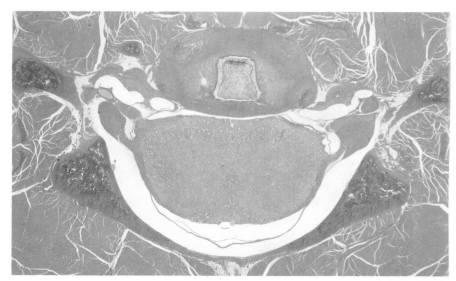

# The brain

Just reading this book is an incredibly complex operation for the brain to handle. It controls the movement of the eyes as they scan each line. It receives from them the pattern of each letter and of the letters in each word, then checks these against the thousands of letters and word patterns stored in the memory. All this happens in a fraction of a second. If you look at an illustration, the brain will interpret the coloured image just as quickly. And all the while, without any difficulty at all, it is registering any sounds that may reach your ears, or perhaps registering the taste of a sweet if you happen to be eating one, as well as controlling such essential functions as breathing, heartbeat and digestion.

Touch your head. It feels quite solid doesn't it? But if the bones of your skull were removed and the brain laid on a table, it would look like a greyish blancmange. Like the rest of the body it contains a lot of water, and being very delicate it has to be protected. It is surrounded by a liquid which absorbs any shock.

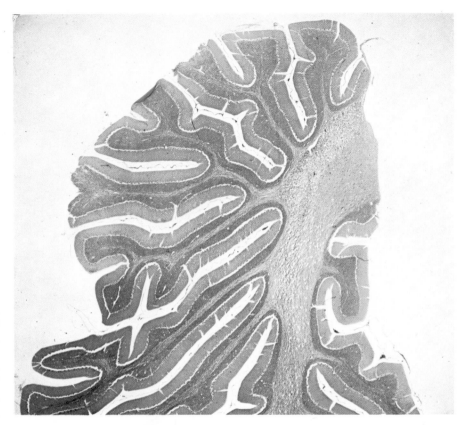

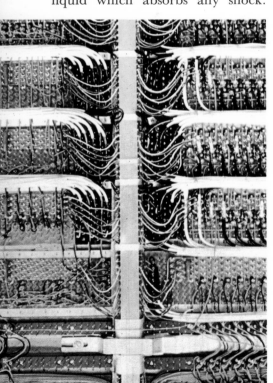

*Above* Cross-section of the part of the human brain known as the cerebellum. The areas shown in orange are the cells which do the brainwork. The darker areas surrounding these are protective tissue.
*Left* Computers are rather like our brains but they are much larger. They can calculate much faster than the brain but they cannot think for themselves and must be programmed.

Covering the liquid is a membrane and this is contained by the skull, which is hard bone. Over the bone is the scalp, which is skin, from which the hair grows. The surface of the brain is not smooth, but wrinkled, rather like a walnut. This gives it a much larger surface area than it would otherwise have, and this is what is so important for intelligence.

If you have seen a new-born baby, you may have noticed that the head is very large in proportion to the rest of the body. At birth your brain probably weighed about 350 g (14 oz). It continued to grow so that by the time you were about six it was nearly full size. An adult's brain weighs just over 1·3 kg (3 lb). Until a baby is eighteen months old the bones in the skull are not fully joined, or fused. On the top of the head is a soft area called the fontanelle, where there isn't any bone at all. It is actually possible to touch the membrane just below the skin. By eighteen months after birth the bones have fused together, making the skull very strong. This bony structure will protect it well under most conditions.

The brain must perform three main functions, receiving information from inside and outside the body, sending out instructions to the glands and muscles of the body, and storing and processing information. It is made up of a number of different parts which are each responsible for certain activities.

At the base of the skull lies the region concerned with balance and coordination known as the cerebellum. Immediately in front of this is situated a small area called the medulla, where groups of nerve cells control the automatic processes of the body such as digestion, breathing and the beating of the heart. It is here too that the spinal cord which conveys messages to the rest of the body's nervous system is connected to the brain. Because the nerves from the spinal cord cross over on their way through the medulla, the left part of the brain controls the right side of the body and vice versa. The left side of the human brain is in fact slightly more developed than the right, which explains why most people are right-handed.

The largest section of the brain is the cortex, which is also called the cerebrum. It takes up 80 per cent of the brain's area. This is the part which you would see if you could look down on a person's brain from above without the skull covering it.

The cortex is the most advanced part of the brain and is responsible for intelligence, memory, thought and all conscious physical or mental activity. It is made up of the grey matter, which consists of a great many nerve cells. The cortex is divided into two areas called hemispheres, each split into four lobes. Since each lobe is connected to the others, it is not particularly easy to say whether one area controls one specific activity. However, through studying the effects of stimulating or removing certain parts, scientists have been able to discover the general functions of the four lobes.

The frontal lobe controls thought and intelligence, mood and behaviour, as well as speech. It also sends messages relating to movement to various parts of the body. The two lobes behind this region are responsible for hearing and memory and for receiving impulses from the body's sense organs. The fourth area is situated at the back of the head and is concerned solely with vision.

Although the hypothalamus is a very small region in comparison with the cortex above it, it has a number of important jobs to do. It is the body's temperature regulator, for by sending out messages it can make a person sweat or shiver. The amount of salt and water present in the blood is something which the hypothalamus also controls. It provides a link between the hormone

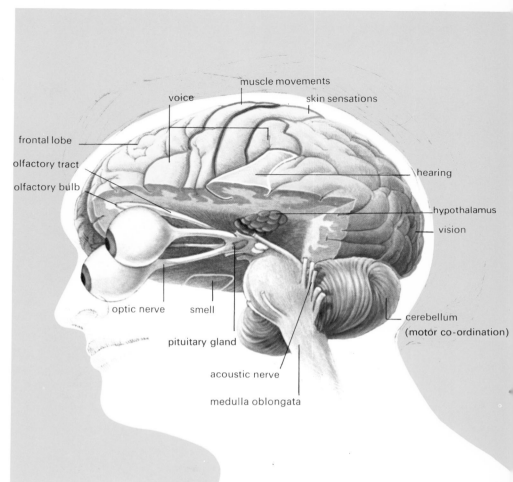

*Above* A diagram of the brain. Part of the upper area of the brain, called the cortex or cerebrum, has been cut away so that some of the other parts are exposed. You will see that various activities are associated with different parts of the cerebrum. Nerve fibres which go from the medulla oblongata connect up with the spinal cord, so that the whole of the body will be served by the nervous system.
*Right* The human brain and its connections with the spinal cord. The vertebrae are small bones which make up the vertebral column, and these protect the spinal cord.

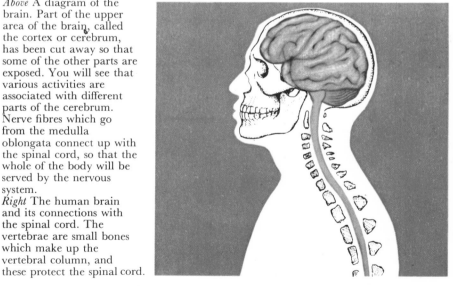

and nervous systems, acting directly on the pituatory gland which controls growth, and is concerned with the regulation of body rhythms and emotions. The thalamus immediately above it receives signals which arrive from the body's sense organs and processes them before passing them to the cortex. Thus the thalamus, can detect pain, for example, but it is the cortex which assesses what sort of pain it is and determines the action which should be taken to relieve it.

# Speech

If you have seen a baby soon after it is born, you will know that the only noises it makes are gurgling and cooing sounds and cries. In fact, until it suddenly finds itself in the outside world at birth, it will not have uttered a sound. If a new-born baby doesn't cry, the midwife will usually slap it to make it cry and start to breathe. During most of the first year of life you would have

They are well placed on top of the windpipe. The vocal cords form part of the voice-box, called the larynx. A person suffering from laryngitis will find it difficult to talk clearly because of an infection of the larynx, caused by a virus.

When the vocal cords are together, they shut the wedge-shaped opening in the larynx. When air is in the windpipe, or trachea, and you

want to breathe out, the vocal cords relax, so that there is a gap between them, allowing air to escape. But air on its own does not make the sounds; we have to do something else. When you speak, muscles in your throat push the vocal cords closer together which makes the gap between the flaps of tissue smaller. Because there is not so much space, these flaps vibrate and produce the sounds. Actually, you can feel the vocal cords vibrating. Put your fingers on your throat on the part which sticks out slightly – the Adam's apple. When you have found it, hum a tune. Do it quietly at first and then gradually increase the sound. Can you feel the vibrations? As you increase the sound, the vibrations get stronger.

There is rather more to the vocal cords than this. You can change the pitch of the voice. Try talking in a high-pitched voice and then in your normal voice. The vocal cords are not loose. At one end they are joined to a piece of cartilage – this is harder material than skin. At the other end there are knobs of cartilage, which are attached to the cords. These

nose cavity

palate

pharynx
tongue
epiglottis

vocal cords

windpipe

spine

*Left* This cutaway section through the head and throat shows the position of the larynx, inside which are the vocal cords. Air comes up the windpipe from the lungs, and as it passes over the vocal cords it makes them vibrate – but only when we want to talk. By changing the shape of the mouth and using the nose and throat we can make the sounds louder. To make different sounds we can move our jaws, lips and tongue. The epiglottis closes the windpipe when we eat so that food doesn't go the wrong way.

made such noises. By the age of one you would probably have learnt at least one or two words. At about two years old children manage to put words together to make simple sentences, and by the age of three most of them will be talking all the time, even if they don't always make sense!

Some children have difficulty learning to speak, and when an infant is born deaf it will usually not learn how to make words because it has never heard any. By the age of four most children can speak almost as well as adults and have quite a large vocabulary.

How is it that we can actually make sounds which we know as speech? You've probably heard of the vocal cords. This is a rather misleading term because they are not really cords at all but flaps of skin. Their position is shown in the diagram of the head on this page.

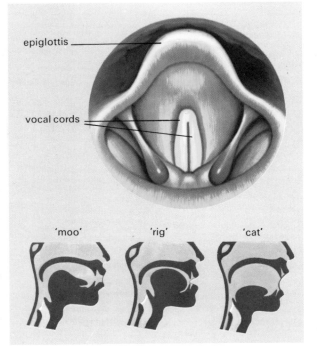

epiglottis

vocal cords

'moo'   'rig'   'cat'

*Left* If we look down the throat at the area of the larynx – the voice-box – we see the vocal cords, which are responsible for the sounds we make. The epiglottis is visible as a flap which will fall over the windpipe. There is a gap between the vocal cords through which air will pass.

*Left* You will see from the three diagrams that the shape of both the mouth and the throat alters when we make different sounds. Say the words shown here in front of a mirror, and notice how the shape of your mouth changes.

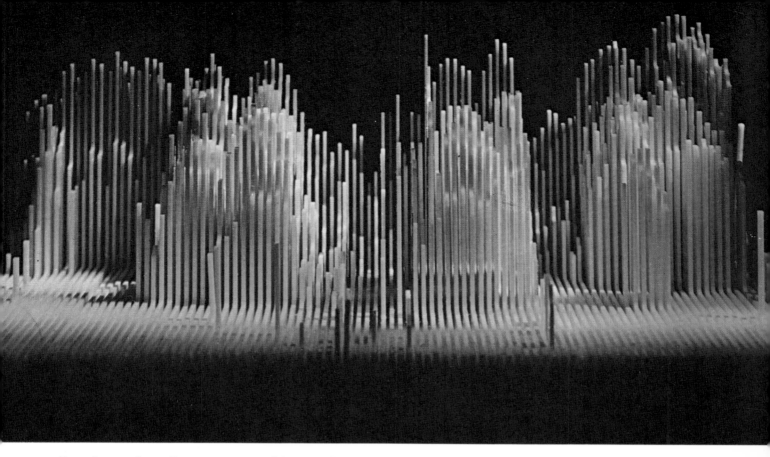

smaller pieces of cartilage are not fixed at the other end and so they can be moved in various directions. When you make a high-pitched sound, the cords have to be tight, and so the knobs of cartilage are tilted backwards, making the cords taut. The opposite happens when you speak in a low-pitched voice, as this slackens the cords. You can see what happens by using an elastic band. Stretch it out and pluck it. What sort of sound did you get? Now slacken it and pluck it. Is the sound different? Tightly stretched bands, or cords, give a high-pitched sound; slacker ones give a low-pitched sound.

It would be difficult to hear the vibrations unless they were amplified. Various parts of the mouth contribute to this. The hard palate—roof of the mouth—as well as the space in the mouth and nose all increase the loudness of the sounds. Try closing your lips and see how much noise you can make, and what words you can say that are loud enough for someone to hear. Unless you are a ventriloquist, you will find it very difficult.

Blindfold yourself and then get some friends—both boys and girls—to talk to you. You should be able to name them because you know their voices. Everybody has a different voice.

When you are young, you will have a higher-pitched voice than when you grow older. As you grow, so does your larynx, and the vocal cords get both thicker and longer. Women's vocal cords are more stretched than those of men, and so they have higher-pitched voices.

Look in the mirror and read the next few lines aloud. What do you notice? The lips move and, although you probably don't notice it, so do your jaws, your tongue and your throat. When you move these, you change the shape of the air space in your mouth, and this changes the sounds.

When you speak, you make the air vibrate. These vibrations, like other sound waves, are collected by the outer flap, the pinna, and directed along the ear channel until they reach the brain. It is the brain which changes the impulses into sounds which we hear. And the whole process of speaking, hearing and understanding takes place so quickly that it seems to us virtually instantaneous.

This is a three-dimensional plastic model of the letters IBM, to represent how they are spoken. Time is represented from left to right, energy vertically, and frequency from front to rear.

# Co-ordination

Have you ever thought how many different actions are required just to ride a bike or run after a football and kick it towards the goal? Getting on the bicycle involves your muscles and your eyes. Once you are on, you will also have to balance, otherwise you will soon fall off. On the football field you will sight the ball, perhaps trap it and then kick it towards the goal, making a judgment as to how far away it is.

In other words, muscles and senses not only have to work well on their own account, they also have to work well together. There has to be co-ordination between them.

In our illustration all the baseball striker wants to do is hit the ball. Quite a simple operation, isn't it? Well, it's not as simple as it seems at first sight. The striker has to have light coming to his eyes so that he will see the ball. He needs other information which comes to his eyes: how far away the ball is, the direction in which it is coming, and where the rest of the players are. While this information goes to the brain, the brain will be working out other factors. The muscles will be sending their signals, giving details of the way in which the body is positioned and how the hands are gripping the bat. Two parts of the brain are involved in what happens. The messages from the eye go to the cerebral cortex (see Brain, page 52). The cortex interprets the information and sends it to the cerebellum. Here the nerves from the senses—eyes, ears and so on—are linked to the nerves which control the way muscles move—the motor nerves. The messages, telling the muscles to act, are passed along the spinal cord. Remember that all this happens very fast and without any conscious effort on our part. We should also remember that in the case of the baseball player the brain won't receive just one set of information—it will have a continuous supply.

Although the information the brain first receives tells it that the ball is in a straight line, it might become obvious as the ball gets nearer that it has changed direction. The brain changes its tactics accordingly. Should all the information received by the brain have been correctly interpreted and the right responses sent back to the body, the striker will hit the ball properly and to a position where there isn't a fielder. Of course, this doesn't always happen, and the ball doesn't always end up where the striker would wish. The judgments which the brain has to make are often difficult ones, but with more and more practice and by using information from past experiences the striker does improve.

Different activities involve a different set, or perhaps more than one set, of muscles. The muscles which the baseball player used to hold the bat and hit the ball will be different from those which he uses when he runs. Muscles cannot work on their own, and so they have to be given

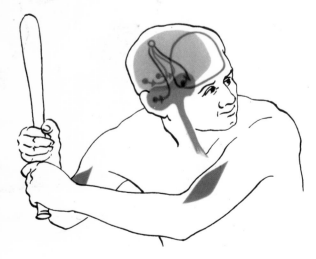

cerebral cortex
cerebellum
to left eye
to right eye

A baseball striker is ready to hit a ball. Both eyes will receive light which will tell how far away the pitcher is, the direction of the ball, and so on. The information is sent to the brain to be sorted out. Receptors in the muscles also send information to the brain about the body's position. The motor centre will tell the muscles whether they need to make adjustments, so that the striker will hit the ball.

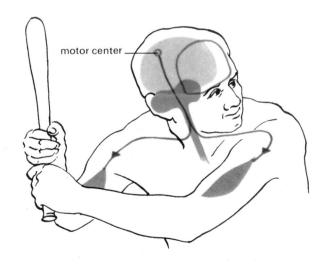

motor center

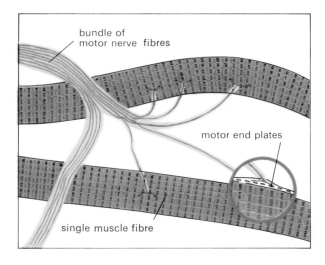

bundle of
motor nerve fibres

motor end plates

single muscle fibre

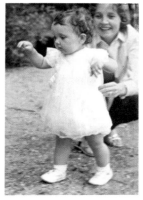

*Above* A baby soon learns to get its balance with help from its parents. At first it falls but it learns from its mistakes, because the brain soon manages to co-ordinate the various activities.

*Above left* Messages from the brain travel to the muscle fibres (brown) along motor nerves (yellow), which are attached to motor end plates. The nerve impulse causes the muscle fibres to contract.

*Left* Some people have better co-ordination than others and can use this to advantage. Improved co-ordination, like that shown by the juggler, will eventually come with much practice.

*Below right* Judo depends on a great deal of co-ordination and relies on split-second changes in balance and pressures. A small man can beat a big one if he has better balance.

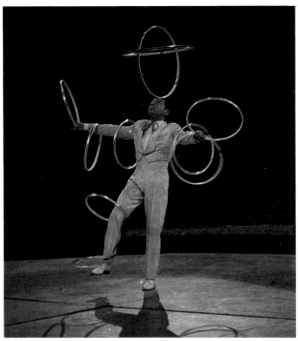

warning other parts of your body to prepare for the crisis. While you were asleep, your heart would be beating quite slowly because you did not need very much energy. But as soon as you woke a hormone, adrenalin, would enter the bloodstream, and the heart would beat faster to get more blood to the muscles. Your breathing rate would also increase to get more oxygen into the bloodstream. In addition, the fire would probably frighten you, and your heart beat would continue to increase. The information about the position of the fire would already have been received, and you would decide how best to escape.

As a young baby you would have had great difficulty in co-ordinating the muscles and nerves. When you first tried to walk you fell over, and continued to do so until you learnt to co-ordinate the muscles properly. Such learning is not confined to infancy or childhood. We improve our skills all the time by building on those we already have.

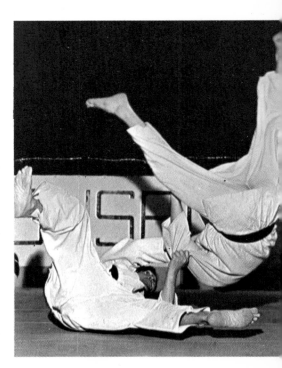

the 'go-ahead': not just when to work but how as well. Each muscle, or set of muscles, will receive impulses via the central nervous system (CNS) which has the correct information. Like other activities in the body, it is the CNS which controls the muscles.

At the moment you are reading this book, but let us say that you have decided to stop because you want to write something down. There's a pencil on the table. You pick it up, but have you ever thought exactly what happens? You will look at the pencil. Your eyes will send impulses to the brain. Information will have to be sent to the various sets of muscles so that

you can actually reach out and pick up the pencil. The shoulder, arm and finger muscles will all be involved.

Let's look at another example. Fire breaks out in your house one night. In a fire there is usually smoke which makes a smell. This would be picked up by the nerve endings in your nose which detect smell. Your ears might also hear the crackling of the flames. The information, passed to the brain, would quickly tell you that something was wrong, and you would wake up. It is likely that as soon as your eyes opened you would see the light caused by the flames, which would tell you the direction of the fire. Already, the brain would be

# Intelligence

The word 'intelligence' is generally used to describe the brain's ability to think, to reason things out, to occupy itself with thoughts and ideas over and above the control and coordination of the body. There is, in fact, still a lot of argument among experts about how intelligence should be defined and measured. All they will usually agree is that intelligence represents what they call the 'highest activities' of the brain. Our ability to receive information, through our eyes, ears and other senses, to store it in the mind and recall it at will—all part of the mental process called memory—is classed as one of these higher activities. Of course, some other animals display intelligence in one form or another, but not, as far as we can tell, to anything like the same degree as ourselves.

If you think about life on this planet for a moment you will soon realize that it is man who is in charge! Although at one time he lived a life much like other animals, wandering across the face of the earth in search of food, his intelligence has developed so that he now dominates the world. The Latin name for man is *homo sapiens*, meaning 'man the wise', though the way we sometimes behave towards one another suggests that we may not always be as wise as we like to think!

People have tried to measure intelligence, and you might even have had an IQ test at school. IQ stands for Intelligence Quotient, and scientists claim that if they give a similar sort of test to different people they can compare one person's intelligence with another's. This doesn't really tell *how* intelligent a person is; it just allows a comparison to be made. Various people have devised tests to measure IQ, and one of the most often used is the Stanford-Binet test. It consists of 'word', 'number' and 'picture' questions. These are chosen to suit children of different ages. For example, most ten-year-olds will be able to answer questions for that age. Some will be able to answer them all; others know the answers for those of eleven-year-olds as well. When a child of a particular age comes to the questions which are too difficult, he has reached his mental age. Let's take a six-year-old. He can answer all the questions for both six-year-olds and seven-year-olds, but none for eight-year-olds. The child therefore has a mental age of seven, and to find his IQ we put the mental age over his real age and multiply by 100. $\frac{7}{6} \times 100 = 116$. The average IQ level is set at 100, so the child is more intelligent for his age. About 75 per cent of the population have IQs which range between 85 and 115. There are people with lower ones, and those who have IQs below 70 need special education because they are slow to learn and understand.

Not everybody does well in the same sorts of tests. If you are good at science, then it is likely that you will

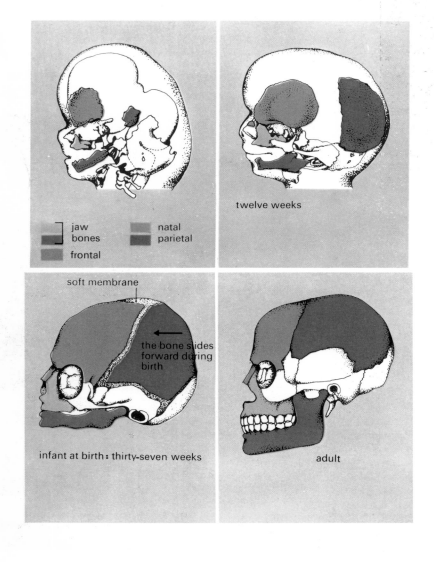

jaw bones

natal parietal

frontal

twelve weeks

soft membrane

the bone slides forward during birth

infant at birth: thirty-seven weeks

adult

Bone growth in the human skull. When the embryo is only 2·5 cm (1 in) long in the womb, the bones have started to grow *(top left)*. At 12 weeks the skull bones are coming into position, so that at birth some will be in place. By the time that adulthood is reached the skull will have changed to its mature form.

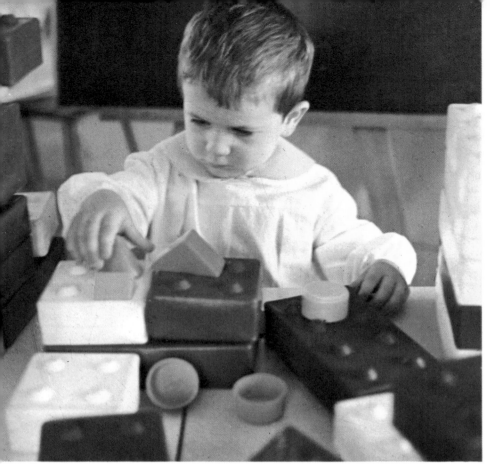

Humans can learn skills like playing the organ or riding a bicycle. Once we have learnt these things, we remember them. Naturally, things don't come all at once, but as we get older we learn to solve more difficult problems, using the knowledge which we already have.

do well in the mathematics part of an intelligence test. On the other hand, you might be artistic, in which case you will almost certainly do better with the pictures. Some of your friends may be better at the parts of the test which involve words, rather than with those which are about figures and pictures. You will see that there are some people who are good at art and not very good at mathematics. You might be one of those people who can deal with figures but who doesn't have a clue about drawing.

Although you might be able to teach a dog to be obedient, this takes a while. Even though he might learn a few tricks, these will be simple ones.

*Above* At your age you would easily fit the right shaped pieces into the correct hole. This three year old has to think very hard about what he is doing. Once he has solved the problem, he will find it easier each time he tries to do it.
*Right* As a child grows it learns to recognize differences in shapes as well as colours.
*Below right* The little girl is reasoning out the way in which the shapes fit together.
*Below left* Differences in a child's abilities to draw an adult: that on the far left is by a three-year-old; that on the right by a child of nine.

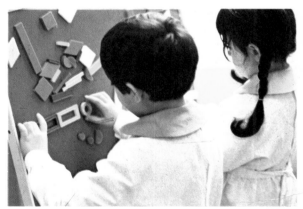

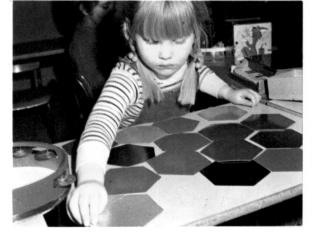

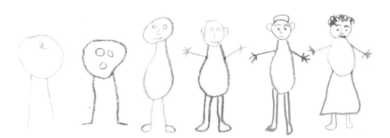

# Chemical messengers

A man has been injured in an accident and he is unable to use his legs. Although he can't walk and he can't feel anything, his leg continues to receive a supply of blood to feed the cells. The nerves which carry messages to and from the leg are no longer functioning, but there is still some contact. In addition to the nervous system in the body there is a second system.

The body produces a number of chemicals, called hormones, which are responsible for making sure that the body works properly. These are the chemical messengers, and it is important that they are able to control the body in times of emergencies, as well as during normal activities. The body has a number of glands, as the illustration shows. The hormones are produced in these glands.

Have you ever wondered why there are a few people who are either very tall—giants—or extremely small —dwarfs? The pituitary gland makes a hormone which controls the way in which we grow. So, unless something has gone wrong with the gland, the chemical which it produces will make sure that you grow to your normal size. But it isn't just growth which the pituitary controls. It has a number of other important jobs to do in our bodies.

In spite of the effect which the chemicals have on the body, the pituitary gland isn't very big. You will see from the illustration that it is found at the base of the skull. Not only does it produce a number of chemicals—it also controls the other glands in the body which produce hormones.

If the pituitary gland makes too much of the growth hormone before a person reaches maturity, then the bones will grow too long, and a taller than normal person will develop. Sometimes the gland doesn't make enough of the chemical, and so instead of growing, the bones never reach their full length, and a shorter than normal person, usually called a dwarf, will result. If there is not enough of this hormone in young babies, they will not grow properly and they may also be mentally retarded.

The drawing shows *some* of the glands in the body. Those, like the sweat glands, control localized bodily functions. The endocrine glands, by contrast, control developments in the body as a whole. They introduce chemicals called hormones directly into the blood. One hormone from the pituitary gland, for example, controls the way in which the body grows during childhood and adolescence, and so the chemical needs to travel to all parts of the body.

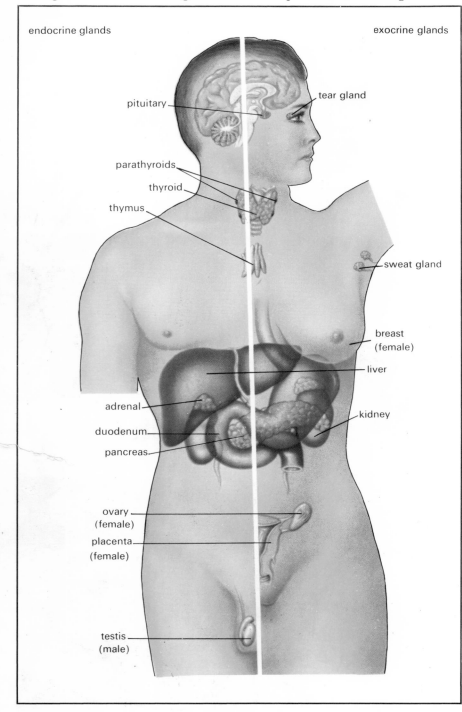

endocrine glands

exocrine glands

pituitary

tear gland

parathyroids

thyroid

thymus

sweat gland

breast (female)

liver

adrenal

duodenum

kidney

pancreas

ovary (female)

placenta (female)

testis (male)

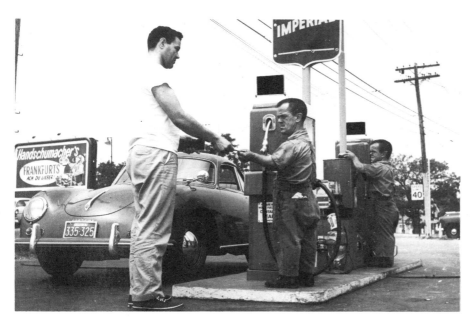

This has happened because another hormone, called adrenalin, has been added to the blood, and this has speeded up various bodily activities.

Hormones also control sexual development and activities. In females the ovaries release chemicals called oestrogen and progesterone which are responsible for such features as the growth of pubic hair and the rounding of the hips and breasts. Progesterone is also important because it ensures that the womb is prepared for a pregnancy if an egg is fertilized (see page 62).

The chemical produced by the thyroid gland is a hormone which makes sure that cells are built up and broken down. It also controls the rate at which the body produces energy. The same hormone, called thyroxine, also controls the way in which the body grows. There is iodine in this hormone, and we usually get this from drinking water. If young babies do not get iodine, they will not grow properly. If older people don't have it, they suffer from a disease called myxoedema. When a person has this, the speech becomes slower, the hair will fall out, and the skin dries and becomes thicker.

Diabetes is quite a common disease in which the body does not produce enough insulin. This chemical controls the level of sugar in the body. Someone suffering from diabetes has to have a regular injection or dose of insulin. If there is not enough insulin glucose cannot be stored for use and the body has to break down fat and protein for energy. When this happens, a lot of acetone is produced, and the body can't deal with it. When it stays in the body, it makes the cells more acid, and eventually the person will fall into a coma. If the person isn't found and the treatment carried out without delay, then he will eventually die.

You've probably been frightened at some time. You know what happens: your heart starts to beat faster.

Dwarfism is not always due to a lack of the growth hormone which the pituitary gland produces. These two people standing beside a normal man, were born dwarfs.

The photograph shows a normal-size man next to a pituitary giant. During his development in childhood too much growth hormone was produced. The result is that the man has grown too tall. In normal-sized people the correct amount of growth hormone—a chemical messenger—is maintained in the bloodstream. Too little of the growth hormone in childhood and adolescence results in very small people, known as dwarfs.

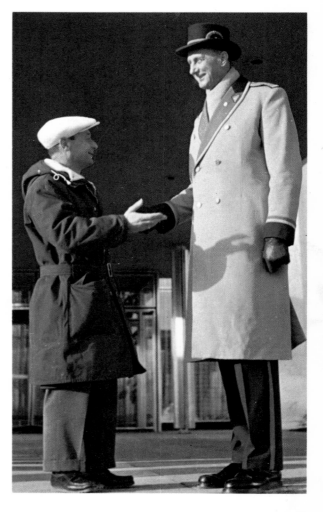

# Start of a new life

Isn't it a wonderful feat that only about forty weeks (nine months) after two very small cells have fused together a baby, with all the characteristics of an adult, albeit in miniature form, is born? All the information necessary for this to take place was carried in those two small cells; information transferred from the parents to the child.

The female reproductive cells (already there when the new child is born) are called ova (singular ovum). The male cells are called sperm. They are not produced until the male child reaches puberty, i.e. the age approaching sexual maturity (about 13 years in a girl, 15 years in a boy). In females the eggs are released at regular intervals; in males sperms can be released at any time. A female egg is released about once a month and if it is not fertilized, it will be discharged. This series of events is called the menstrual cycle (commonly known as the period). At roughly monthly intervals chemical messengers will be released by the body. These will start the cycle of events. The egg in the ovary will start to develop. This

goes on for about twelve days. Other parts of the body are also prepared. Once the egg has been released from the ovary, it drops into the fallopian tube and could be fertilized. The womb starts to thicken, which is a means of preparing itself to receive the egg. Once the egg has been released it travels down the fallopian tube on its way to the womb. If sperm meets it within forty-eight hours of its departure, the two will fuse together. The egg will travel to the womb where it will start to develop. Each month a female from about the age of thirteen to fifty or so, releases an egg.

It is necessary for the sperm to get to the egg. These male cells are produced in the testes, contained in the scrotum, a small bag of skin which hangs outside the body underneath the penis. Millions of sperm cells are produced regularly, and it is necessary for the penis to be inserted into the vagina of the female. Normally, the male organ hangs limply outside the body, but when the male is aroused it increases in size and becomes stiff, or erect. It can then be inserted into the vagina.

By a series of up-and-down movements the man stimulates the sperm to move along the tube by a series of muscular contractions until they emerge at the end of the penis.

The release of the sperm cells is known as ejaculation. Large numbers are necessary because very few will complete the journey to meet and fertilize the egg. The sperm cells are rather like tadpoles, and their long tails help them to swim into the fallopian tubes. It may be that the sperms were released at a time when there wasn't an egg ready to be fertilized, in which case they will die. Of the many millions which set off on the journey perhaps a hundred or so will arrive at their destination. Even though there may be an egg, the sperms may not fertilize it, and the embryo will not start to develop.

Once a sperm has managed to penetrate the wall of the egg, fertilization has taken place. The tail part falls off, and the head area gets bigger. The sperm continues to push into the egg until it reaches the nucleus in the centre. Once the ovum and sperm have joined, the

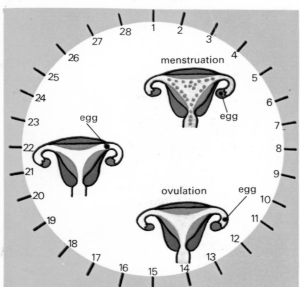

*Above* If an egg is not fertilized, menstruation will take place. Part of the lining of the womb will be discarded along with some blood.

*Right* Although the embryo is only nine weeks old and measures 40 mm, it already looks like a miniature human being. A sac of fluid in the womb helps to protect the embryo.

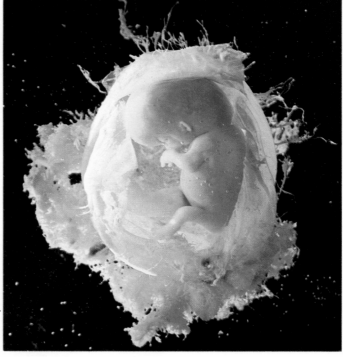

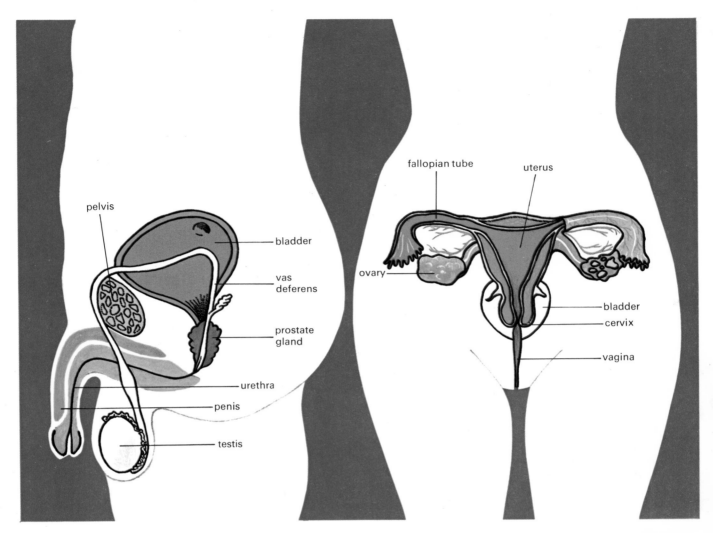

pelvis

bladder

vas deferens

prostate gland

urethra

penis

testis

fallopian tube

uterus

ovary

bladder

cervix

vagina

new offspring will start to develop. The new cells will have a full set of chromosomes: twenty-three from the ovum and twenty-three from the sperm. When the cells have joined, they form a new cell called the zygote, and conception has taken place.

No more sperm are needed, but they might try to push their way into the egg. To prevent this the outside of the zygote becomes harder, so that other sperms cannot enter and those which are not needed will die. Fertilization is the start of a long series of events which will result in the birth of a baby (see page 64).

Sometimes a fertilized egg will divide into two parts, and in this case twins will develop from the same egg. When this happens, they will be identical. Moreover, there are two fallopian tubes and these release an egg alternatively: one comes from the left tube one month,

and from the right tube the next month. Sometimes two eggs are released. If both are fertilized, then twins may again develop. These twins will not be identical because they have come from two different eggs. From time to time triplets may be born, and even quads and quins.

Men and women do not necessarily want to create a new life every time they have sexual intercourse, in which case they must prevent the sperm coming into contact with an egg if one is there. There are various ways of ensuring this. The man can cover his penis with a thin rubber covering, called a sheath. This collects the sperm when they are ejaculated. Alternatively, the male may take his penis out of the female's vagina before he ejaculates so that sperm are not released inside her body. It is possible for the woman to stop eggs being released from the ovaries by taking a con-

In the male the liquid semen containing the sperm is released through the penis. In the female the egg (ovum) leaves the ovary and travels down the fallopian tube. If a sperm meets an egg and fertilizes it, a baby will develop.

traceptive pill. In other cases the female may have her fallopian tubes cut, which also prevents the eggs coming down. The male may have his vas deferens, the tubes which carry the sperm, cut and tied so that sperm are not released. This is called a vasectomy.

# A baby is born

At conception the ovum and sperm cells came together. About a day later the zygote, as it is now called, will divide into two. Although the sperm and the ovum were very different in appearance, the two new cells which are formed are alike. The zygote is still in the fallopian tube and it will divide yet again before it starts the journey to the womb. Once it has reached the uterus, it will become attached to the wall. When this happens, the process is known as implantation. Scientists are not really sure how this happens. It could be that a small hole has been made in the wall of the uterus, or the embryo might make a hole for itself. This will happen between five and seven days after the cells first joined at fertilization.

Although nine months might seem a long while from the time of conception to birth, the zygote has got to change into a baby. Many of the organs in the body form quite early in the pregnancy. In most cases the heart inside the foetus will be beating after twenty-five days. When X-rays have been taken after eight weeks, the embryo actually looks like a miniature version of a human being. It will have a mouth, eyes and ears. The limbs can be seen, and the toes are already formed. But it will still be less than 4 cm (1½ in) long, which is only about the same length as two of the joints on the finger of an adult's hand.

Each of the various parts of the body which we can see—the ears, arms, and so on—start off as buds in the foetus. As the cells continue to divide, so the complete parts, like the ear, appear, and fingers can be seen on the end of each hand. The first limb buds appear twenty-six

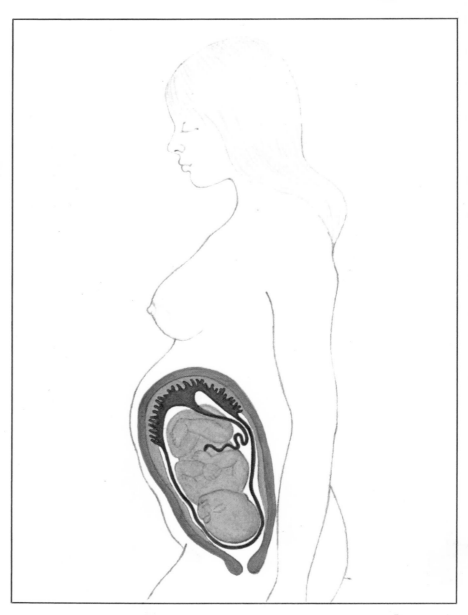

*Above* A baby developing in the womb. Before it is born, it should be in the head-down position. The umbilical cord linking the mother and the baby can be seen. *Below* With the baby's head in the correct position a birth will usually be straightforward. During the birth contractions of the uterus and the muscles of the abdominal wall and pelvic floor push the baby out.

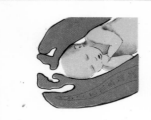 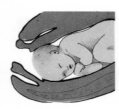 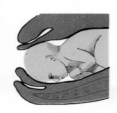 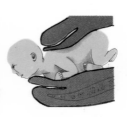 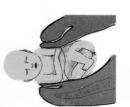

days after fertilization, and on the thirty-third day the outline of the fingers can be seen. Although during the tenth week the pregnancy is one quarter of the way through, the foetus will have to increase its weight *six hundred* times before it is due to be born.

To make sure that it is protected the foetus floats in a liquid sac. So that feeding can take place there is a pipe, the umbilical cord, which joins the growing foetus to the mother. Although the baby needs to be fed by the mother and to have waste products taken away, there is a barrier between the two. This is the placenta, and it stops the mother's blood from mixing with that of the foetus. Substances needed by the developing infant can go through the placenta, and these include oxygen and food. The mother's blood will have antibodies in it (see page 75), and these also go through the placenta to the blood of the foetus.

When a baby is ready to be born, labour will usually start on its own. No one really knows what makes labour start. Sometimes it is possible to start labour artificially by giving drugs to the mother. With normal labour there are three stages, and although these may differ slightly, most happen in the following way. In the first stage the uterus or womb starts to contract. To begin with there will usually be a long gap between each contraction, perhaps twenty or thirty minutes. Gradually they take place more frequently until there are only two or three minutes between each one. This stage of labour will go on for about fifteen hours or so in the case of the mother's first pregnancy. It doesn't always last so long with the next and subsequent pregnancies. The second stage then starts, and this is the actual birth. Gradually the muscles help to push the baby along the uterus towards the vagina. How long this stage lasts varies from a few minutes to several hours with a first baby. The head is the first part to appear, and this is usually followed quite quickly by the rest of the body. The placenta and membranes are discharged in the third stage which lasts about twenty minutes.

Although most births take place

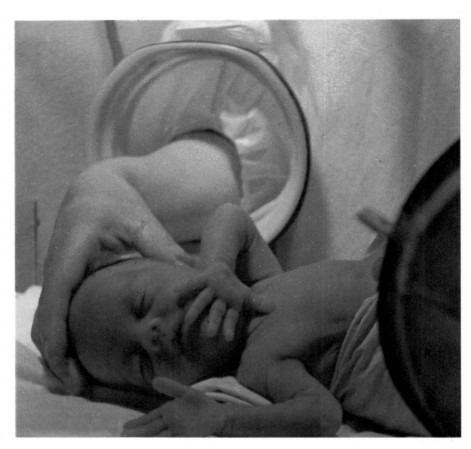

normally, sometimes problems do arise. The head may not be in the downward position and the baby is still curled up so that the bottom comes out first. Sometimes, too, there is a risk that the umbilical cord may be twisted round the baby's neck. When there is any danger to either the baby or the mother, or perhaps to both, it may be necessary to cut the abdomen wall and remove the baby this way. This is known as a Caesarean birth.

When premature babies are born (perhaps four or five weeks ahead of time) they often have to be taken to an intensive care unit and placed in an incubator until they have gained in strength. Even a baby born at the normal completion of a pregnancy may have various defects. Perhaps it cannot breathe properly, or it has something wrong with its heart. There may be a defect like a damaged spine, in which case the child may be paralysed. All these problems will be dealt with in the intensive care unit in a hospital, so that the baby will have the maximum amount of care and attention and can be watched constantly.

If a baby is born too soon, then special attention may be necessary. This baby has been placed in an incubator. Here it will be kept warm and protected from germs which might make it ill.

# Growing up

During the nine months in the womb the embryo or foetus has grown until it is fully developed and ready to be born. In the safety of the womb it has received all it needs through the lifeline attached to its mother: the umbilical cord. Although its heart has been beating and pumping blood around its body, its lungs have not been used. It has got the necessary oxygen from the mother. Now at birth all this has changed. The baby is ready to lead an independent life. The umbilical cord is cut after birth, because the new-born baby's body will need to survive on its own. The lungs have not been used and they are filled with liquid, but during birth the fluid is squeezed out of them, preparing them for their first intake of air. It is believed that mild asphyxiation stimulates that part of the baby's breathing, and so the baby takes its first vital breath.

The new-born baby seems ready to lead an independent life of its own. But this isn't strictly so, as you will realize. A new-born baby, although it can breathe and its heart is beating, is very much dependent on its parents for the first years of its life. A new mother will produce milk in the breasts which she will use to feed her baby. Not all mothers produce enough milk or are able to feed their offspring. Artificial milks containing all the nutrients of a mother's milk will be used instead. The baby has to be fed, it has to have its nappy changed, and it must be protected.

See if you can find a photograph of yourself as a baby and then as a young child. Then look in the mirror so that you can see what has happened to you over the years. Look at the pictures of a child growing up on this page, and you can see what changes take place.

When you were born, you were not able to walk. This was because the bones of your body weren't rigid, and other parts of your body, including the brain, were not sufficiently developed to co-ordinate muscle and eye movements. Can you think why it might be a good idea to have soft bones at birth? It makes the actual birth easier, because the hard bones could get damaged on the way from the womb to the outside world. They could also damage the mother as well. You will also recall (page 15) that the bones of the skull were not joined together at birth. In fact, bones do not start off by being made up of bone cells, but from cartilage. Over a period of time this is replaced by bone cells which make the limbs harder and more versatile.

If you think about it, you will soon realize that there are lots of things a baby cannot do which we take for granted. It can't control its movements; it isn't able to focus its eyes and see things properly. All these aspects will improve as the baby continues to grow. There are some things, however, which the new-born baby must do to stay alive.

*Below* For the first nine months of life the foetus develops inside the womb of the mother. For the first few months after birth—it varies from about six months in some babies to a year in others—the child will feed on either its mother's or artificial milk. For the first four months or so it can digest only liquids. From four months it starts on solids. For the first year at least it needs a great deal of help from its parents. As it grows, it develops its own balance so that it can walk, and to some extent it becomes independent, although it still relies on its parents.

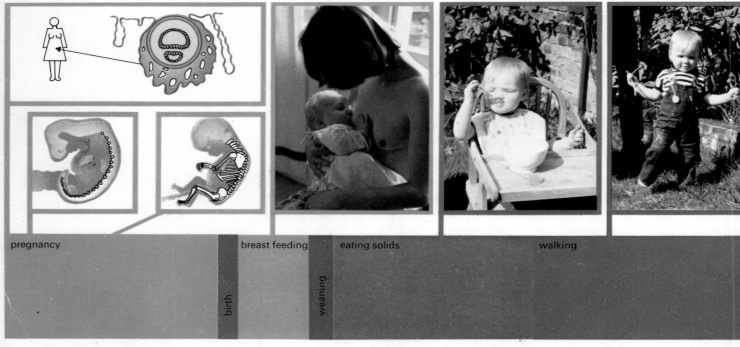

pregnancy   breast feeding   eating solids   walking

birth   weaning

0   9   0   3   4   12   mo

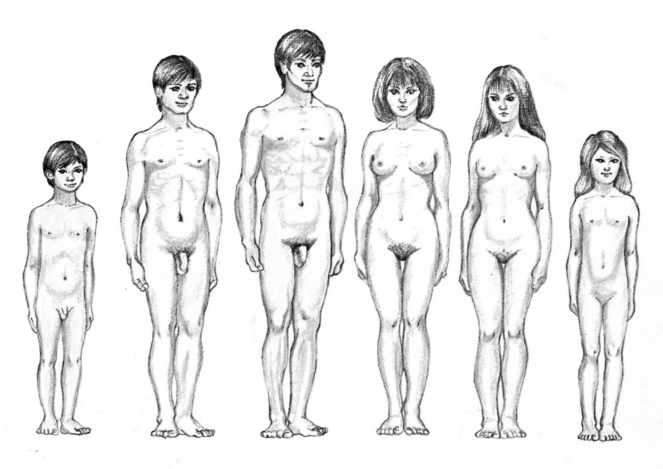

The baby has to be able to suck—either its mother's nipple or the teat on a feeding-bottle. Once it has the food in its mouth, it needs to swallow it. These are important for its survival, but there are numerous other things which it must learn to do—balancing, talking, walking, and so on.

Gradually, over the years the body grows, and the greatest period of change takes place at puberty, which is a part of adolescence. It is difficult to give an average age, but girls start to develop sexual characteristics from the age of about ten and boys from about twelve years. Girls' hips start to get wider, and the menstrual cycle will begin its monthly activities. The production of one of the sex hormones, called oestrogen, stimulates certain activities. Hair will grow in the genital region as well as under the arms. Breasts increase in size. The shape of the body will change slightly, so that it takes on a more rounded female appearance.

In boys the sex hormone testosterone will be released. This stimulates certain activities, and hair will begin to grow in the genital area, under the arms and on the face. Here it is soft at first but it gradually becomes bristly. The voice will break and change from a high pitch to a lower one. At the same time the sex organs will grow more rapidly. Both the penis and the testes will increase in size, and sperm will start to be produced. It is not unusual for growth to take place quickly, making a boy tall and clumsy-looking until his muscles develop. Growth usually stops by about the age of twenty-one.

*Above* As a person grows up not only do the bones get longer, so that height increases, but sexual characteristics develop. In the male the sex organs increase in size, and hair develops in the pubic region, on the face and under the arms. In girls the body takes on a more rounded shape. The breasts increase in size, and hair appears in the pubic region and under the arms. In early childhood the shape of boys' and girls' bodies was much alike; by about the age of fifteen the differences are quite marked.

Changes are taking place inside the body as well. Chemical messengers (hormones) will be released to make sure that sperms will be made and eggs released.

# Why you are you

Take a look at the patterns on your fingertips. The way in which those curves, whorls and circles are formed by the ridges of skin is absolutely unique to you. Everybody else's fingertip patterns are unique as well, which is why police forces all over the world use fingerprints as sure proof of a person's identity.

Fingerprints are only one of very many ways in which we are all different from each other. Indeed, many of these differences are far more apparent than fingerprints. We are tall or short, fat or thin, blue-, brown-, or grey-eyed, dark-haired or fair-haired, go bald early or keep our hair till the day we die. Beyond matters of appearance there are such features as the sound of our voice, the way we generally behave, the things we are good at doing and the things we find difficult to do. All these features, of physical appearance, of manner and behaviour, and of ability, combine to make each one of us unique.

The factors that determine all these things about us are found within the nuclei of our body cells. (See Cell, page 8). The nucleus of each cell contains minute, thread-like substances called chromosomes. There are forty-six of these in each nucleus, arranged as twenty-three pairs. These chromosomes, in their turn, are made up of chains of particles called genes, of which there may be more than a thousand in a single chromosome. Genes are composed of a complicated chemical called deoxyribonucleic acid, or DNA. Sugar, phosphoric acid and what are called four bases—adenine, cytosine, guanine and thymine—are the ingredients of DNA. The molecules of these substances arrange themselves rather like a spiral ladder within each gene. The bases, linked in special combinations, as though they were the rungs of the ladder, are the factors which actually hold the key to our whole appearance and personality.

Our genes are not something we create within ourselves. They are the material of inheritance. When someone says we have our mother's eyes or our father's smile, they are commenting upon the way the genes of one parent or the other have been passed on to us and so influenced some particular feature, expression or manner of our own. This inheritance is established at the moment of conception, when the male sperm cell fertilizes the female egg cell. Each of these special reproductive cells contains twenty-three chromosomes, which combine to form the required forty-six chromosomes in the cells of the new life.

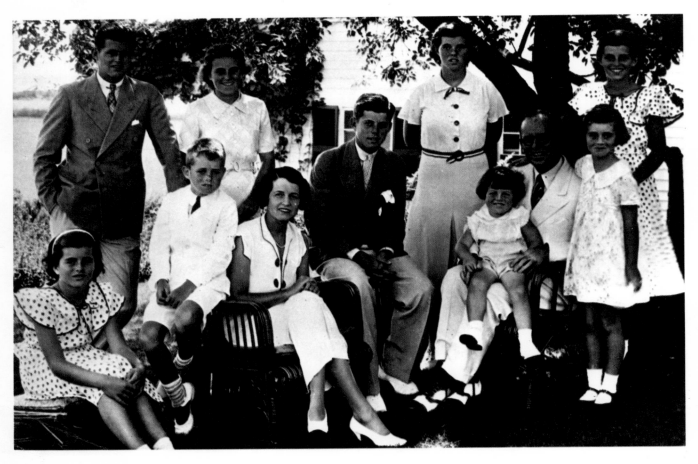

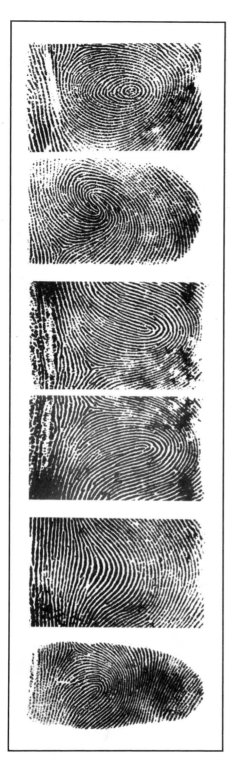

The above six fingerprints are all different from each other. Everybody's fingerprints are unique, even those of identical twins. In the past they were often used on official documents in place of a person's signature. They have long been used by the police to establish a person's identity. *Opposite* Group photograph of the Kennedy family showing very clearly the way in which physical features are shared by closely related people.

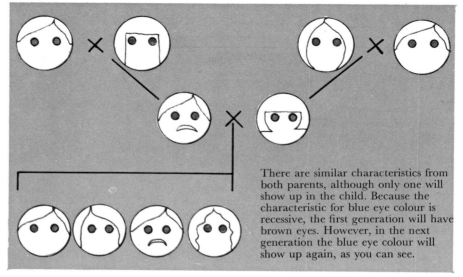

There are similar characteristics from both parents, although only one will show up in the child. Because the characteristic for blue eye colour is recessive, the first generation will have brown eyes. However, in the next generation the blue eye colour will show up again, as you can see.

The most fundamental thing to be determined is that of the sex of the newly evolving life, and the way this is done provides one example of how genes and chromosomes form up to make us what we are. All male cells contain one pair of chromosomes consisting of one Y-shaped and one X-shaped chromosome; while female cells all have one pair of chromosomes which are both X-shaped. The sex of the individual is decided at conception by whether the Y-chromosome in the male sperm cell combines with one of the X-chromosomes in the female egg (producing a boy), or whether it is the X-chromosome in the male sperm which combines with one of the X-chromosomes in the egg (producing a girl). Thus it is from the moment of conception the genes and chromosomes form a pattern that determines the sex and everything else about the newly created individual. It is a pattern that is repeated and conveyed, like a coded message, to every other cell of that individual, from the time when he or she is still growing in the womb, right through life and up to death.

Genes give their name to the science of genetics, the study of the way that certain features are handed down through reproduction from one generation to the next; and the way these features can sometimes disappear in one generation, only to appear again in one or more members of succeeding generations. The illustration on this page shows how the colour of eyes is determined according to the matching up of genes inherited from previous generations. This matter of dominant and recessive genes, as explained in the illustration, applies to many other features. Unfortunately, it also applies to certain physical weaknesses or diseases. Haemophilia, for example, is an inherited disease, carried by females but affecting males only. The genes responsible for this condition of the blood may pass harmless through the genetic make-up of many members of a family, only to regain dominance in one unlucky son.

The case of identical twins, that is twins with the same genetic make-up, is very interesting. They are created when a female egg has already been fertilized by a male sperm and then divides to form two separate embryos, each of which continues to develop in the womb as a separate baby. What also sometimes happens is that the mother produces two egg cells instead of the normal one. If both are fertilized at the same time by sperm cells twins will again result, though in such cases they will grow up to be as different as ordinary brothers and sisters.

# Growing old

Our bodies are rather like clothes. They will gradually wear out. As with garments, some parts may wear out before others. When the process of growing old starts is difficult to say. Some people suggest that certain body functions are at their peak at birth. Healing of wounds is an example of this. A cut will repair itself more quickly when a baby is born that at the age of two or three. Actually, we don't notice this change because it is very slow. It's the same with most of the body functions, like the process of ageing. It doesn't happen overnight but takes place gradually.

Apart from the period in the womb, which is the greatest growth period in the life of a human, the next spectacular period of growth is during adolescence. Once growth is completed, the process of ageing will start. No matter what we do about it we know that once we are born so must we eventually die.

You can look at a person and tell whether they are young or old, especially by the appearance of their face. No doubt you will decide that the woman in the picture is very old, because of the heavy lines and wrinkles on her face. But significant signs of ageing will exist inside her body as well.

According to the Bible the average age is 'three score years and ten', which is seventy. Of course, that was supposed to apply to people thousands of years ago, but even today it remains about the average age. However, whether this age in Biblical times was anything like seventy seems doubtful, since the death rate among infants and children was so high. Today, thanks to medical care and a better diet, most people do survive birth and infancy and live to see their seventieth birthday.

The bones in the body will grow for the first twenty years or so of life, and by this stage they will have reached their maximum length. Then they start to deteriorate. In some people deterioration will be more rapid than in others. If you look at the two X-rays, you will see that in osteoarthritis (see page 86) the space between the joints of the bones of the finger is much less than that in the three-year-old boy.

Scientists can't give an exact date at which something will go wrong in our bodies. The way things wear out or go wrong varies from person to person. In one the eyesight may start to fail earlier than in another. Somebody else may find that his hearing has diminished before his eyesight. If it were possible to compare a number of people of the same age, say sixty, it is likely that they would have aged in different ways. One might have poor hearing, another might not be able to see as well, and so on. Some people tend to age less quickly than others.

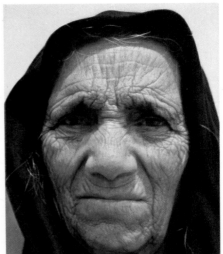

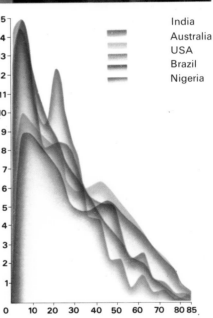

India
Australia
USA
Brazil
Nigeria

*Above (Top)* It is possible to tell an old person from a young one because of the wrinkled skin. *(Bottom)* Fewer people reach old age in poorer countries than in richer nations.

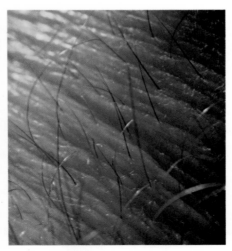

*Left* The two photographs of the skin show many differences between that of a young person *(far left)* and that of an old person *(near left)*. The skin in a young person is smooth and without wrinkles. As a person gets older, the skin becomes wrinkled and lined, and is no longer stretched tightly. It does not look so pink because of changes in the blood supply. It is not unusual for hair to start to grow on the faces of women, but in most cases this can be removed.

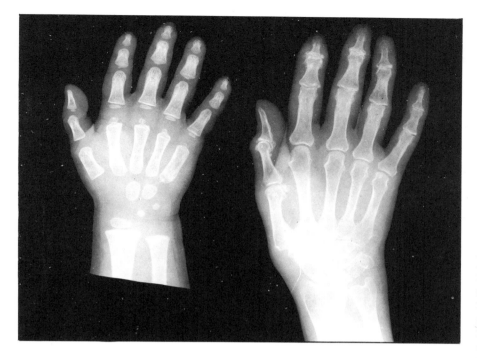

grows clouded. With modern surgery it is possible to replace many of these defective parts (see page 88).

Some of the cells in the body die off at regular intervals, as you can see from the chart. As a person gets older, the replacements become fewer and fewer, and so the body becomes less efficient. The number of nerve cells which help us to find out what is going on around us, as well as carrying messages to and from the brain, start to die off. Because no new ones are being made, the body becomes less sensitive. This is true of the senses of feeling, tasting and smelling, as well as those of seeing and hearing. The result is that people are not able to do things which they could when they were younger. You will notice that in very energetic sports like football the players are not usually more than thirty years of age. Most are in their twenties. See if you can find out the ages of your nearest football league club players. It would also be interesting to see whether the youngest—and, supposedly, the fittest—are found in the top divisions rather than in the bottom ones. As they get older, footballers are not able to cope with the strain, although they probably still train regularly, and as a result of the decrease in their nerve cells, their reactions are not as quick as they were when they were younger.

In women the ability to produce babies stops at the menopause, when no more ova are released. This varies from one female to another but usually occurs at about fifty. Although the number of sperm produced by the male decreases as he gets older, most men are able to father children until they are quite old, but the precise age varies from one male to another.

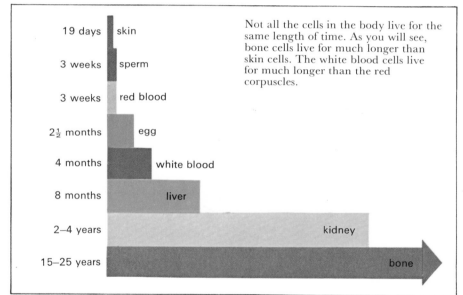

| | |
|---|---|
| 19 days | skin |
| 3 weeks | sperm |
| 3 weeks | red blood |
| 2½ months | egg |
| 4 months | white blood |
| 8 months | liver |
| 2–4 years | kidney |
| 15–25 years | bone |

Not all the cells in the body live for the same length of time. As you will see, bone cells live for much longer than skin cells. The white blood cells live for much longer than the red corpuscles.

As a person gets older, parts of the body change. When this happens on the outside of the body, we can observe it quite clearly. The hair starts to turn grey and may eventually go white. In men it may fall out and cause baldness. If a man had a father who went bald, then the chances of his doing so are greater than for someone whose father kept his hair. Baldness does not seem to start at any particular age. In some men hair will start to fall out while they are in their twenties; in others it is later.

Around the face and neck the skin

which was once smooth becomes wrinkled and often it will take on a more dull and rather lifeless appearance.

We have already mentioned that the eyesight changes, and this varies with different people. Sometimes the lens doesn't remain clear, which means that the person will not be able to see so well. The muscles attached to the lens do not work as well as they did, and so the shape of the lens can't be changed. The cornea, the transparent covering over the front of the eye, won't let light through so easily, because it

# Hair and nails

In other mammals their coat of hair protects them from the cold and the wet. Our own ancestors also grew hair over most parts of their body. Hair is less important to us because we wear clothes and have other ways of protecting ourselves from the elements.

Where do you think your own hair grows the quickest? It is probably on your head, though in male adults it is the beard which grows just a little more quickly. The hair in a man's beard grows about 0·38 mm each day, and the hair on his head at 0·33 mm a day. As people get older, the hair doesn't grow quite so quickly, but during an average person's lifetime it grows about 8 m (25 ft). By this time next year your hair will have grown 12 cm (4¾ in).

If you have a magnifying glass, have a look at the hair growing on your arm. You will see that the hairs don't grow evenly over the surface, and it's the same on the head. The hair grows in clusters with a particular pattern.

How does our hair grow? Cells in the skin form a little pocket, called a follicle, inside which the root of the hair grows. If you pull a hair out of your head – do it quickly and it won't hurt – you will see there is a bulge at the end where it was growing out of the head. If you have a magnifier, you should be able to see this more easily. The only part of the hair which is growing is the root. Because it is growing it needs to be fed, so it has a supply of blood which brings food. The hair is lubricated by glands which supply oil to the follicle. This stops the hair from becoming brittle and breaking easily. Each hair lives for between two and four years. Every day some hair falls out, and new hair grows.

You will have heard people say that their hair stood on end when they had a frightening experience. Hair can stand up because there is a muscle attached to the follicle at the root end of the hair. If the muscle contracts, the hair will stand upright.

If you look around you, either in your own house or at school, you will see people with different-coloured hair. Like eye colour (page 69), we also inherit the colour of our hair. The pigment which gives hair its natural colour is added to each cell at the root. You've probably noticed that as people get older, their hair changes colour, because the pigment is no longer being made. A person doesn't usually go grey or white overnight; it is a gradual process.

As with hair, so nails, or claws, are more important to other animals

Magnified cross-section of the skin showing the way the hair grows.

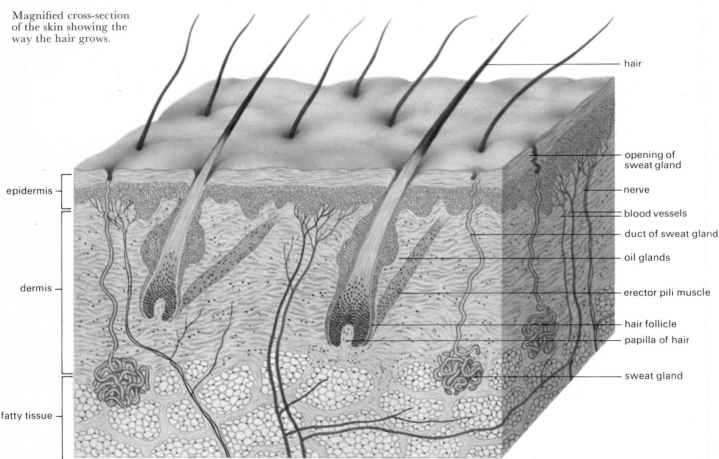

epidermis

dermis

fatty tissue

hair

opening of sweat gland

nerve

blood vessels

duct of sweat gland

oil glands

erector pili muscle

hair follicle

papilla of hair

sweat gland

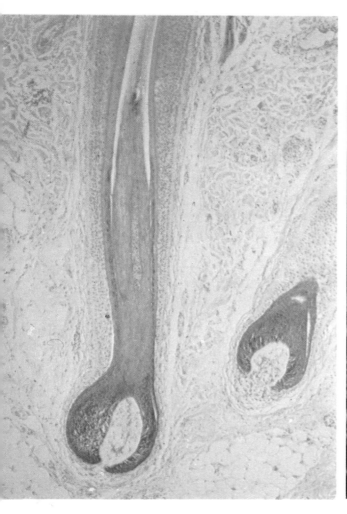

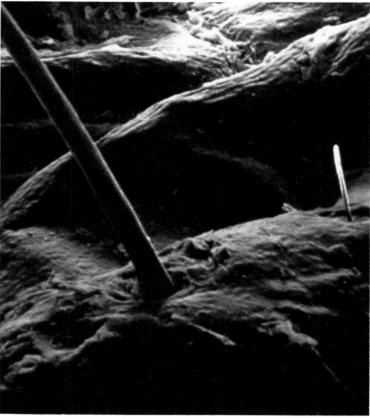

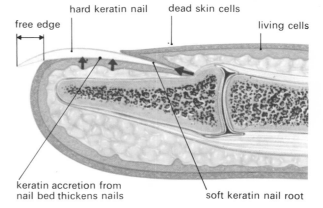

*Above* This magnified section of a piece of human skin shows the make up of the hair root. Hollow at the bottom, it is supplied with blood which will bring food and take away waste.
*Above right* Photograph taken through an electron microscope shows the hairs which grow from the surface of the skin. You can also see that when the skin is magnified it is not smooth.

*Right* Nails grow from the top layer of the skin. Nail cells have keratin in them which makes them hard. The growing part of the nail is the area where it is joined to the skin. We don't feel anything when we cut or break the end off the nail, because this part is dead and does not have nerves. It hurts only when we pull the living part away from the root.

hard keratin nail    dead skin cells

free edge    living cells

keratin accretion from
nail bed thickens nails    soft keratin nail root

than to ourselves. But we were born with nail buds, and most of us will soon start to grow strong, healthy nails to protect the tips of our fingers and toes.

You will see that there is a difference between the skin and nails, although both are made from cells. The difference is that the cells in the nails have a horny substance, keratin, added to them.

Like the hair, nails grow from the base, where they are attached to the bone by connective tissue. The part which you can see and which you cut is dead. If you have lost a nail at some time, it has probably grown again. New nails will grow as long as the root is still alive. A complete new nail will take several months to grow, at the rate of about 1 mm $\left(\frac{1}{25} \text{ in}\right)$ each week. As new cells are added at the base of the nail, they push the rest of it forward.

The doctor may look at a person's nails, and from these he can sometimes tell if something is wrong in the body. If he finds that all the nails on the hands are spoon-shaped, this may be a sign of anaemia—lack of sufficient red blood cells. Sometimes other temporary upsets occur in the body, and white spots, cracks or channels may appear in the nails. They may be caused by pneumonia, for example, but they will usually disappear as the nail continues to grow.

73

# Dealing with disease

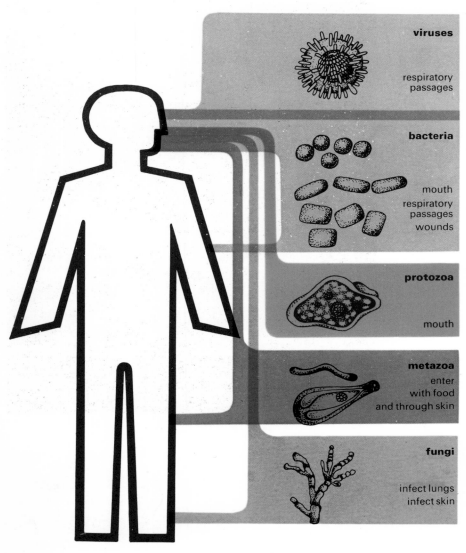

viruses
respiratory passages

bacteria
mouth
respiratory passages
wounds

protozoa
mouth

metazoa
enter with food and through skin

fungi
infect lungs
infect skin

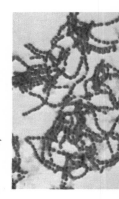

*Left* The body is constantly under attack from all kinds of organisms. You will see that there are various ways in which they can get into the body. The main means of entry is through the mouth. They may be breathed in with the air or taken in with unclean food. Others enter through wounds in the skin. Usually, the body's defence system is able to deal with these. There are times when it is not able to do this, and it may be necessary to take pills or medicines supplied by a doctor. These contain chemicals to attack the invaders.
*Above right* These germs (magnified 1,000 times) cause throat complaints.

Have you had a cold lately? Although you probably felt quite poorly for a while, with a runny nose and sore throat, it wouldn't have been long before the cold disappeared. Have you ever wondered how it is that you get a cold in the first place and then how you get rid of it?

There are minute living things in the air around us. These include bacteria, protozoa and fungi. Both Pasteur and van Leeuwenhoek could see them only under the powerful lenses of their microscopes. Because bacteria and viruses are so small and because there are so many

different sorts, we know of the existence of only some of them. However, scientists have found that different bacteria cause different diseases. Tonsillitis is caused by a different bacterium from the one which causes a boil.

There are also different ways in which such organisms enter the body. Some of them will get in through the mouth, others through wounds, and yet more through the nose. Bacteria may also be in our food and get into the body this way. There are some which attack the skin itself rather than enter the body.

We are surrounded all the while

by organisms which cause disease, and some of them will be constantly entering our bodies. When a disease-causing bacterium or virus gets into the body, it finds an ideal situation. There is warmth and plenty of food. Let us see exactly what happens when a bacterium enters through a wound in the skin. Very quickly it increases in numbers and produces toxins. These are poisons which go into the blood and will be carried round the body. The toxins affect the body, while the bacteria continue to reproduce in great numbers. If this continued, it would not be very long before the bacteria took over the body and the person died.

Fortunately, the body has a good defence system which will go a long way to repel the invaders. You will remember that we have white cells in the blood, and some kinds of these, called phagocytes, become active. They will arrive at the site of the invasion ready to attack the bacteria. These organisms are much smaller than the white cells. Very soon the phagocytes will engulf and digest the bacteria. Other white cells, called lymphocytes, make and release their own chemicals. These are called antibodies, and they fight the toxins making them harmless.

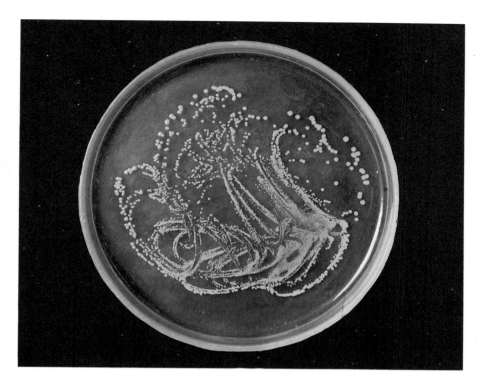

Bacteria streaked on to a plate of jelly containing food will grow. For example, a sample of urine may contain several different types of bacteria. Each will form a colony which can be transferred to another plate to grow and be studied further.

The lymphocytes are made in the lymph nodes, which are found in the tonsils and adenoids. As the bacteria come into the body, the tonsils and adenoids help to filter them out. When the body is under attack, the tonsils swell because they are producing many lymphocytes to kill off the invaders. Have you had your tonsils out? They are often removed because when they swell they can become very painful. Our bodies can manage without them because we have other means of defence.

To find out which particular bacteria cause which disease scientists cultivate them in the laboratory. Using small plates of a special jelly, they streak the surface with bacteria. Because the jelly has food in it, the bacteria will grow and reproduce.

How quickly do the bacteria reproduce? If there is enough food and the temperature is right, then each will divide every twenty minutes. Within an hour there are eight, after two hours sixty-four and after seven hours no fewer than two million bacteria. It was a German scientist, Robert Koch (1843–1910), who first saw bacteria grow into colonies. Scientists have found that all the bacteria they have seen can be divided into three groups according to their shape. Some are spiral (like a corkscrew), others are cylinder-shaped, and yet more are almost round. Some of the spiral bacteria have tails; some of the cylinder-shaped bacteria have hairs. These extra parts help bacteria to move.

Without regular food and water you would soon die. However, some bacteria have a means of surviving when conditions are not very favourable. They form structures called spores. Inside the cell a watertight capsule develops, enclosing all the vital parts of the cell. The cell wall breaks down after a time, leaving the spore. The spore can survive extreme heat and cold and is so light that it can easily be carried on currents of air. Bacteria can survive in this form for many years, and when conditions are again favourable they can start to reproduce.

Foot-and-mouth disease is a serious illness among cattle, but not among humans. The germs of this disease can enter our bodies, but we have what is called immunity to them. In other words, before the invaders make us ill, white cells in the body have dealt with them. We call this type of immunity 'natural immunity'. When you were developing in your mother's womb, her blood passed on the natural immunity to certain diseases.

*Left* A doctor examines a child's throat for signs of infection. He may take a sample of mucus containing bacteria on a swab, so that he can grow these to find out the cause of the illness.
*Right Diplococcus pneumonia* (magnified 1,000 times), a bacterium causing bacterial pneumonia.

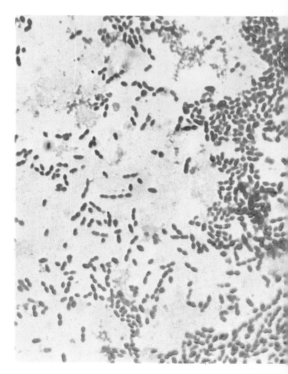

Have you heard of smallpox? You might have, but few people catch it now. If you had lived in earlier times, you might have suffered. Edward Jenner was a doctor from Gloucestershire who lived from 1749 to 1823. He saw many people who either died or were badly scarred as a result of catching the disease. He believed that people who suffered from a similar disease called cowpox did not get smallpox. To find out whether this was so Jenner decided to inject a small boy with some of the pus from a cowpox sore. To give the boy cowpox the doctor scratched the surface of his skin and applied some pus.

The boy was soon feeling poorly from the attack of cowpox but he recovered. Now the doctor had to decide whether to give the boy some smallpox germs to see if the cowpox had produced immunity. This he eventually did, after much heart-searching, and to his relief the boy did not get smallpox. This was the first successful vaccination against smallpox. Until recently every child was vaccinated against the disease, but since it has now died out in most countries children no longer need to be protected.

You will be able to see how immunity works from the diagram on this page. The antigen, which is a foreign body to the blood, will make the blood produce antibodies, which will soon destroy the antigen. Next time the actual germ enters, the body will be able to make the antibodies quickly and so destroy the invaders. Bacteria used for immunization are either killed or modified so that they can no longer cause the disease, but can still protect by stimulating the white blood cells to produce antibodies.

On some occasions antitoxins are injected into the blood, and these will attack the toxin. Diphtheria used to be very dangerous, and many people died from it. It was found that if the toxin from diph-

## how immunity works

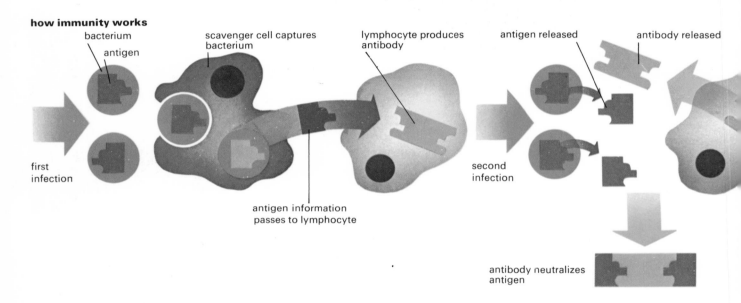

bacterium
antigen
scavenger cell captures bacterium
lymphocyte produces antibody
antigen released
antibody released
first infection
antigen information passes to lymphocyte
second infection
antibody neutralizes antigen

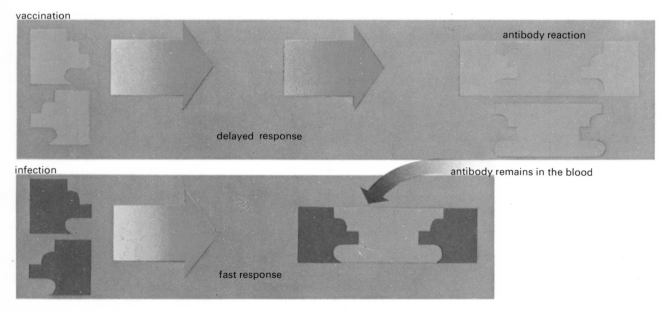

vaccination
antibody reaction
delayed response
infection
antibody remains in the blood
fast response

theria was injected into a horse, the animal would quickly produce antitoxins without getting the disease. The antitoxins could then be taken from the horse and given to a person with diphtheria. Nowadays antitoxins are taken from a person who has recovered from the disease, and given in injections. Fortunately, other vaccines can help to protect us from various diseases, like poliomyelitis, and whooping cough.

Many discoveries have been made by accident. You will probably have heard of penicillin and might even have been given an injection, but do you know how this was discovered? Professor Alexander Fleming was interested in the bacteria which caused boils, and in 1928 he was growing some bacteria in his laboratory. While he was away for a few days, one of the lids came off his dishes. When he returned and looked at this dish, he noticed there was a blue-green mould growing around the bacteria. When he looked more closely, Fleming found that where the mould was growing all the bacteria had been killed. The mould had produced some substance which had gone on to the dish, attacked the bacteria and stopped them from growing. He called his substance *penicillin* after the mould which had produced it. Substances, like penicillin, which stop bacteria from growing are called antibiotics.

Not only are medicines and drugs used to deal with disease, but it may be necessary to use other methods. Cancer is very difficult to cure, and radiotherapy may be used to kill the cancerous cells. Great care has to be taken so that healthy cells are not killed as well.

*Top left* When a disease-carrying organism enters the body, scavenger cells in the blood engulf it. This takes time and the body may show signs of disease. Meanwhile the white cells (lymphocytes) produce antibodies which neutralize the poison (antigens) made by the bacteria. If the same type of bacteria enter the body a second time, the white cells will know which antibody to release – the body is now immune.
*Left* A vaccine contains a disease organism that has been made harmless, but still carries its antigen. The body will then react to the injection by making antibodies. When attacked by the actual organism the body will quickly respond by producing the right antibody.

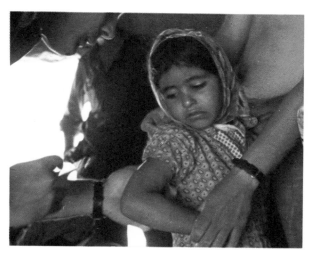

In the poorer countries diseases which have disappeared elsewhere still kill many thousands of people every year. This Arab girl is receiving a vaccine so that her body will build up an immunity to certain diseases which will prevent her from catching them.

Two types of fungi are growing on this culture plate. The darker of the two is a mould known as *Penicillium*. It is from this mould that the antibiotic penicillin, discovered by Alexander Fleming in 1928, is made. It can be used to treat many diseases, although there are people who are allergic to it. The light-coloured growth is known as *Aspergillus*.

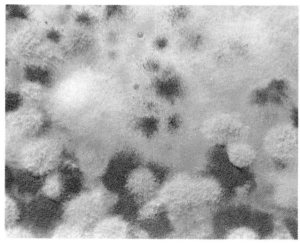

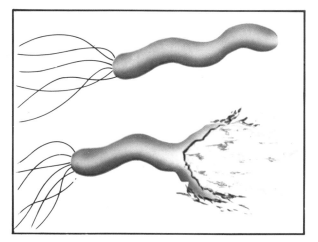

The drawings of the two bacteria illustrate the difference between a healthy, and therefore dangerous, one, and one which has been treated with an antibiotic. The top one is healthy, but the bottom one has been attacked because an antibiotic has been given to the person. One of the ways in which these substances work is to attack the cell walls, which break down so that the contents are set free. These are then carried in the blood and will be eliminated because they are poisonous.

# History and discovery

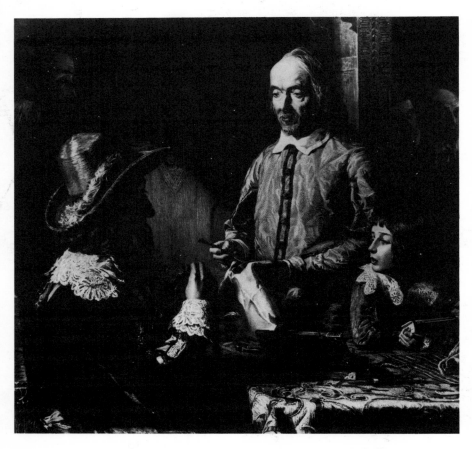

William Harvey made a great impression with his discovery of the circulation of the blood. Here he shows a heart to King Charles I and explains how blood is pumped round the body.

Today we know a great deal about the way our bodies work. You can read that the heart pumps blood round the body and that there are veins and arteries. But how did we find out about these things?

About eighteen hundred years ago a Greek physician (doctor), named Galen, wrote about medicine. For hundreds of years students read his books and believed that what was written in them was true. Some of the information was correct, but much was inaccurate. For about fourteen hundred years people used Galen's writings. Even though he had probably not been able to look at a heart, he said that there were invisible holes in the central wall. Blood with air in it was thought to pass through these holes from one side of the heart to the other. Then people had other ideas. Servetus, a Spanish physician, said that there were no pores but that the blood went through the lungs. In 1571 an Italian, Andrea Cesalpino, went further and suggested that blood actually circulated round the body.

William Harvey, an English physician, considered further the idea of circulation. He cut up hearts and looked at the blood vessels in human beings. He agreed with Cesalpino. One of the intriguing things which he discovered was that there were valves in the heart, and because of the way in which they were arranged blood could go in only one direction.

Harvey did some experiments using humans. Earlier people had said that the blood flowed back-wards and forwards rather like the tide on the seashore. Harvey tied off an artery and stopped the blood from flowing. Behind the place where he tied the artery, on the heart side, the blood collected and formed a bulge. When he tied a vein, he found that the blood collected on the side of the binding away from the heart. He suggested that the blood in the arteries flowed from the heart and blood in the veins flowed to the heart.

Harvey then went on to look at how the heart worked. He found that the amount of blood which went through the heart in 60 minutes was three times the weight of an average man. He realized that this was a colossal amount. If an average man weighs 72·7 kg (160 lb) this means that 218 kg (480 lb) of blood goes round the body every 60 minutes.

Harvey wrote down his discoveries, and these were printed in a very important book called *Exercitatio de Motu Cordis et Sanguinis*, which translated means 'On the motions of the heart and blood'. Although this was only 52 pages long, it contained Harvey's carefully recorded observations. As well as looking at humans, Harvey studied frogs, fish, snakes, and he even looked at the heart of a chick still developing inside the egg.

Although Harvey discovered the arteries and veins and said that the blood circulated, he did not write about capillaries, the very small tubes which make sure that the blood is taken from the arteries to every cell and returned via the veins.

Anton van Leeuwenhoek (1632–1723) was a Dutchman who found that if he ground glass down into lenses he could magnify things. He made some simple microscopes using a single ground glass lens. Leeuwenhoek watched small insects as they developed. He looked at drops of rainwater and saw in them tiny organisms. These animalcules, as he called them, were too small to be seen by the naked eye. He watched the life cycle of very small animals, including fleas. He saw

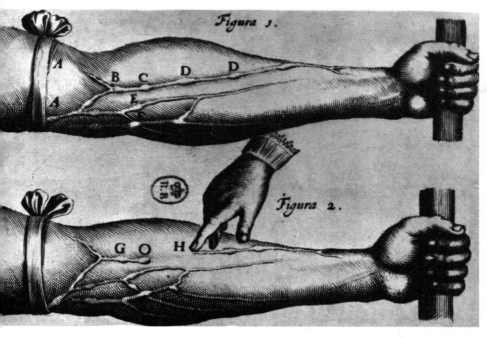

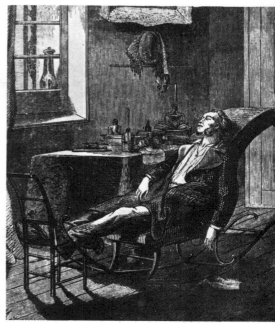

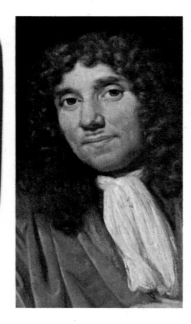

*Above* The work which William Harvey did was published in book form in 1628. Not only did he write about his investigations but he included many illustrations. In the two figures Harvey shows how blood collects in the forearm when a bandage is tied around the veins. By doing this Harvey was able to state that blood in the veins flowed to the heart.

*Above right* Charles Jackson, an early experimenter, tried the effects of ether on himself.

*Far right* Anton van Leeuwenhoek produced his own microscopes to look at small organisms. Although he did not actually invent the instrument, he did much to increase the magnifying powers. He was able to look at a wide range of organisms.

*Right* Each of Leeuwenhoek's microscopes had a screw which moved the object up and down. The sharp needle held the object he was looking at. The single lens was placed between two metal plates.

both the eggs and the larvae of ants. Looking at the eyes of insects, he was the first man to observe that their eyes were made up not of one lens but of many lenses. He also looked at sperm cells.

The Italian biologist Marcello Malpighi had already discovered the capillaries which Harvey had overlooked. Leeuwenhoek viewed the blood system of tadpoles and not only did he see the very small blood vessels but also the blood cells. By careful and dedicated study the Dutchman also managed to draw

the shape of muscle cells directly from the microscope.

Leeuwenhoek's microscopes were surprisingly powerful because he discovered other very small creatures which he had great difficulty in drawing. These turned out to be bacteria. With this information the French chemist Louis Pasteur was able to link bacteria and disease.

Until the middle of the last century, if anyone had to go into hospital for an operation, they were fully conscious while the surgeon was operating. Just imagine having a leg off or your appendix out while able to feel the whole thing. In spite of the fact that a good surgeon could remove a limb in less than a minute, the person still suffered agonies of pain. Then a surgeon, William Morton, working in America, demonstrated the use of ether gas which he used as a general anaesthetic. By placing a mask over the patient's face the gas would be breathed and would soon send him to sleep. At about the same time as Morton was doing his work in America James Simpson was trying out chloroform gas in Scotland for the same purpose.

We are lucky living in the 20th century because if we are ill we will usually recover thanks to the attention of doctors and nurses. Behind the scenes other people are carrying

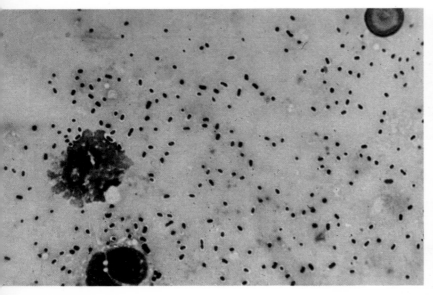

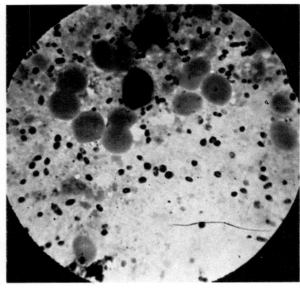

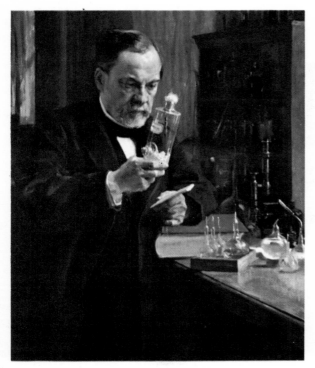

*Above* The two bacteria shown in the illustrations were named after Pasteur. The one on the left is called *Pasteurella pseudotuberculosis*. Although it affects other animals, it seldom attacks humans. The other *(top right)* is *Pasteurella pestis,* the bacterium which causes plague. It was quite common up until the 18th century and caused countless deaths throughout Europe. Fleas and infected black rats were largely responsible for outbreaks of the plague.

*Left* Louis Pasteur started his work by looking at wine and later turned his attention to diseases affecting animals. He discovered that bacteria made things go bad, which caused disease.

out valuable research into various diseases and trying to find new cures.

We have already seen how Harvey discovered the circulation of the blood and how Leeuwenhoek discovered bacteria. Then came Pasteur, one of the greatest scientists of all time.

Louis Pasteur, born in France in 1822, trained as a chemist, but it is for his work in the fields of biology and medicine that we remember him best. Pasteur's early work was with wine and beer. He took samples of both good and bad wine and looked at them under the microscope. If your parents make wine or beer at home, you will probably know that they use yeast in it. Yeast cells are living, and when yeast is added to sugar and grapes it feeds on the sugar. During the feeding a chemical process called fermentation takes place and alcohol is produced.

When Pasteur looked at good wine, he saw round yeast cells. When he looked at bad wine, he saw rod-shaped cells. These cells did not make alcohol; instead they produced lactic acid which turned the wine sour.

Pasteur decided to heat the wine for a few minutes to a temperature of 55°C, (131°F), which killed the cells, and fermentation stopped. As long as the wine was bottled and corked securely, bacteria could not enter and the wine did not go sour. This method of heating liquids, like wine and milk, to stop them from going bad is called pasteurization.

Pasteur then turned his attention to silkworms. Using his earlier research, he found that one insect could pass on a disease to another, and realized that bacteria were involved. More significantly he identified the presence of these 'germs' in the air. After Pasteur made it clear that this was how disease was caused, doctors started to boil their instruments and to use disinfectants to kill off the bacteria.

Turning his attention to other problems, Pasteur decided to heat the bacteria which cause anthrax in the same way that he had heated the wine. He found that although the heat did not actually kill the bacteria it made them less dangerous. He now injected the heated bacteria into animals. Because the bacteria were not so dangerous, the animals suffered from only a mild attack of anthrax. To kill off the bacteria the animal's body produced antibodies. If the animal came into contact with the disease again, the antibodies still in the blood killed off the bacteria. You have probably benefited from

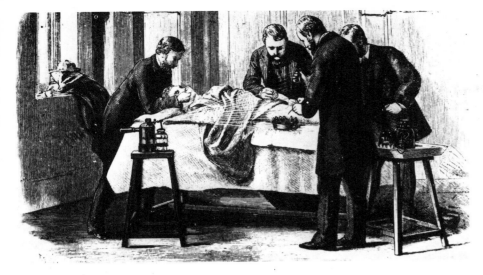

Pasteur's work in this field when you have been vaccinated.

Pasteur then turned his attention to the disease known as rabies. When a dog suffering from rabies bites a person, the virus from the dog gets into the victim's bloodstream. Eventually, the central nervous system will be attacked, and death will usually result.

In 1885 Pasteur discovered a small boy who had been bitten by a rabid dog. Taking a chance, Pasteur vaccinated the boy, who did not suffer from the effects of the disease. Pasteur's vaccine was then used many times to save people from the terrible effects of rabies, although it remains a dangerous disease.

If you went into hospital to have your tonsils out, you would soon be home again. A hundred years ago this would not have been so. The chances are that you would have died. Joseph Lister set about trying to make operations safer. As a surgeon in Edinburgh, he noticed that many wounds often became inflamed. The wounds did not heal but got worse and often led to the patient's death.

Lister became interested in Pasteur's work. He thought that the wounds probably went 'bad' for the same reason as the wine. He already knew that carbolic acid (phenol) would kill simple forms of life, and so he decided to use this on the wounds. After experimenting for a while, he found that the phenol worked. Bacteria in the air were getting on to and then into the wounds. He used the donkey engine shown on this page to spray his operating theatre and kill the germs.

When a wound goes bad, it is said to be septic. The substances which Lister used were antiseptics. 'Anti' means 'against', and 'sepsis' means 'decay', so you can see how we get the word. But in spite of his discoveries, Lister did not realize that clothes, hands, and even water had bacteria in them. Nowadays everything used in an operation is sterilized.

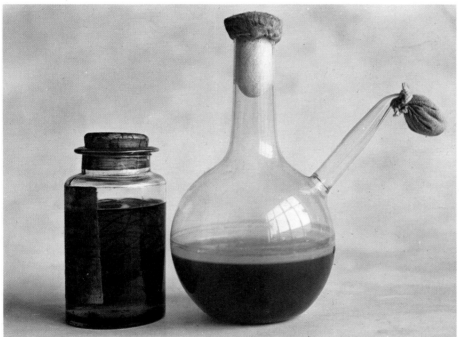

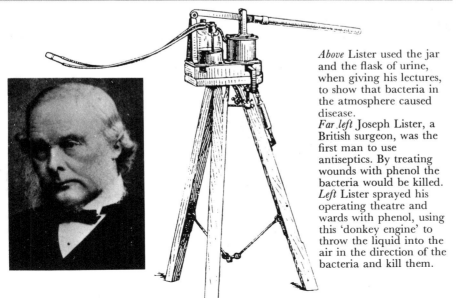

*Above* Lister used the jar and the flask of urine, when giving his lectures, to show that bacteria in the atmosphere caused disease.
*Far left* Joseph Lister, a British surgeon, was the first man to use antiseptics. By treating wounds with phenol the bacteria would be killed.
*Left* Lister sprayed his operating theatre and wards with phenol, using this 'donkey engine' to throw the liquid into the air in the direction of the bacteria and kill them.

# Hospitals

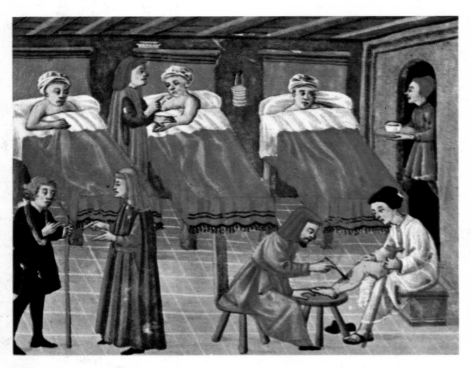

Interior of a 15th-century European hospital. There were both in-patients and out-patients departments. People who were able to attend the hospital came regularly for treatment. Others were kept in.

What do you think of when the word 'hospital' is mentioned – perhaps an ambulance rushing up with some injured person inside? Although the emergency service is very important in saving lives, there are many other things which go on in a hospital. You might go to hospital to have your tonsils removed, or you might break a leg and have to have it put in plaster. Your mother might go to the maternity department to have another baby.

Modern hospitals are very busy places, very different from those of the past. When the ancient Egyptians were ill, they relied on the help of the gods and slept in their temples. This was in 4000 BC (that's nearly 6,000 years ago). Instead of having doctors the ancient Greeks relied on the priests to look after them. But in those days anyone who suffered from diseases was thought to have done something wrong. The gods were important to earlier peoples. Since their illnesses were supposed to be caused by evil, they had to ask the gods to help them.

Not everybody in the ancient world accepted these beliefs.

Hippocrates was one of the greatest of the earlier teachers of medicine. It is not surprising that he soon became known as the 'father of medicine'. He ran his own school of medicine on the Island of Cos. Here he used diet and exercise to help cure his patients.

Many early hospitals were set up by the church as places where blind and crippled people, as well as those suffering from leprosy, could find sanctuary. One of the first hospitals of this kind was St Bartholomew's in London. It was founded in 1123, and is still one of our most famous hospitals.

There were two early types of doctors working in hospitals; physicians and surgeons. As time went by, the surgeons stayed in the hospitals, while the physicians opened 'surgeries' in their own houses. As better hospitals were established, particularly in Europe in the 17th century, they became important as medical schools. Here students came to learn so that they could go out and practise on their own.

Most modern hospitals have two main departments – out-patients and in-patients. The out-patients department deals with people who do not need to stay in hospital for treatment. Hospitals hold clinics where people can attend regularly if, for example, they need to do regular exercises for a damaged leg or a shattered arm.

Unlike the family doctor, the hospital doctor has much more equipment which he can use to discover diseases. If you have a simple illness, your family doctor will be able to treat it. If he can't, then he will send you to the hospital for further tests. Once these are complete a report will be sent back to your doctor.

Modern hospitals are equipped to deal with almost every kind of illness or accident. If you should ever have to go to hospital you might well be sent to the pathological laboratory for a blood or urine test, or to have X-ray pictures taken of certain parts

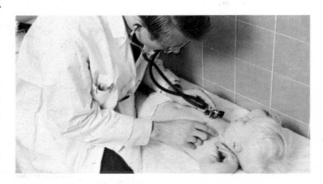

*Left* A doctor listening to a child's heart to discover whether there are any signs of disease.
*Opposite* Ambulances are often equipped with modern devices, whereby emergency action can be taken. This is important since people are often transferred from one hospital to another for operations which are urgent.

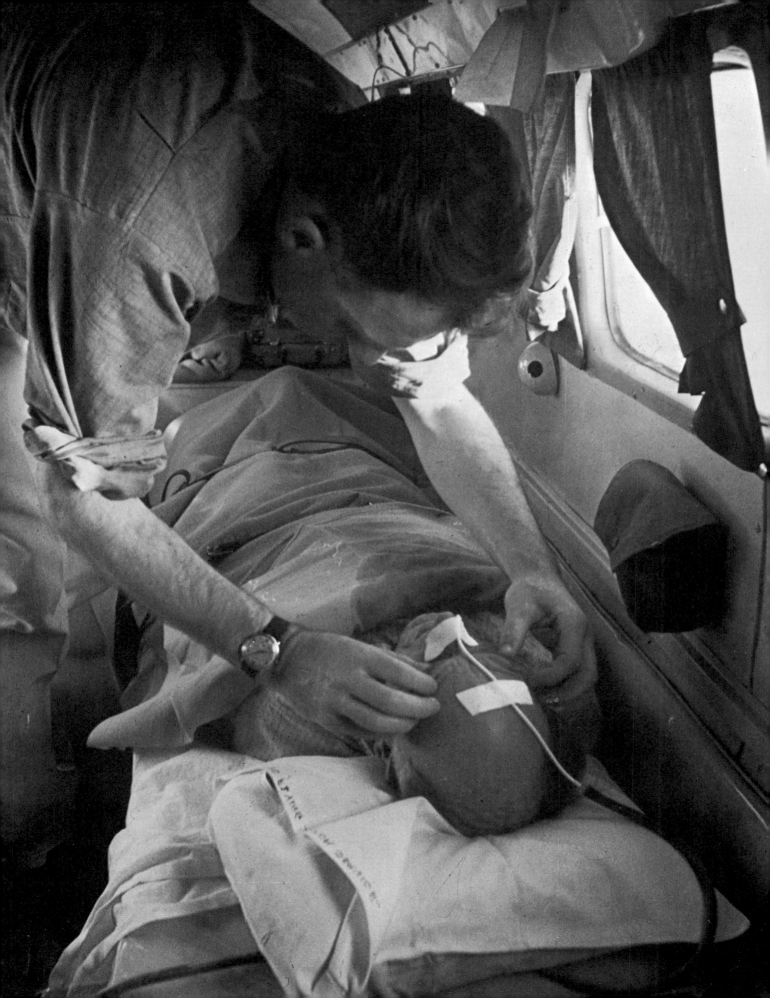

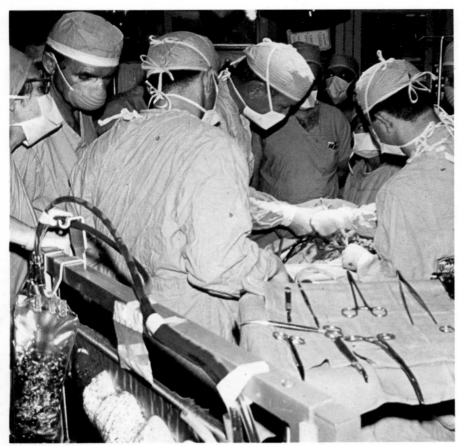

of your body. If you had to remain in hospital for any length of time you'd probably be sent to the hospital dentist as a matter of routine. It would all be part of the service which is provided.

Hospital staff must always be ready to deal with emergencies. They have to be ready 24 hours a day to receive accident cases and to have the patient in the operating theatre within minutes of arrival. Indeed, some hospitals have mobile units, like the one shown on this page. Such units can go straight to the scene of an accident, conduct X-ray examinations and blood transfusions on the spot, even perform an emergency operation prior to the patient's arrival in hospital.

Hospital doctors also hold clinics where out-patients can attend regularly for certain types of therapy—treatment designed to get the patient's body thoroughly ac-

*Left* A team of doctors is working on a patient's diseased heart. As well as putting things right, doctors are also concerned with preventing diseases. This they do by using modern methods to detect disease in its early stages.

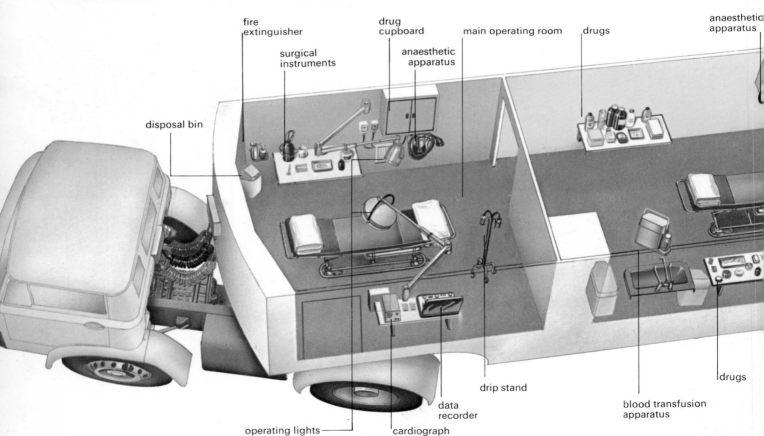

fire extinguisher

drug cupboard

main operating room

drugs

anaesthetic apparatus

surgical instruments

anaesthetic apparatus

disposal bin

drip stand

data recorder

drugs

operating lights

cardiograph

blood transfusion apparatus

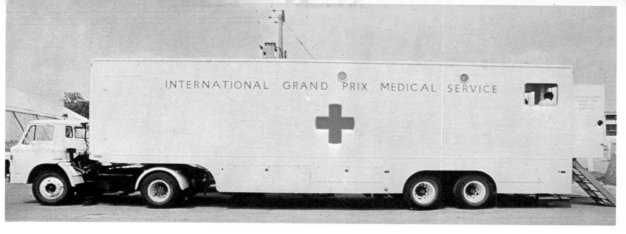

A mobile hospital unit is able to carry the equipment necessary to deal with almost any emergency.

customed to normal life again after hospital treatment.

Some patients need the attention of two or three specialists. For example, someone involved in a serious car accident will have any broken bones set by one doctor. Another will attend to his cuts and other lacerations. A third may have to perform plastic surgery–perhaps reshape a part of the patient's face if it has been badly disfigured. And if his legs are badly damaged, he may have to learn to walk again, which will be the job of highly-trained physiotherapists.

There are plenty of other people in attendance at hospitals who are not doctors or nurses. Patients often need advice from social or welfare departments; or they need welfare workers to look after their families while they are sick and out of action. Children in hospital for any length of time need teachers to give them lessons. Others again provide patients with such services as mobile libraries.

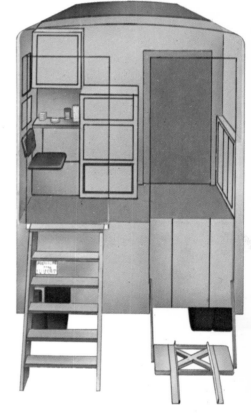

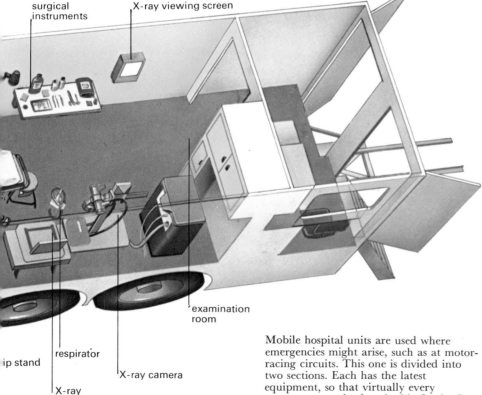

surgical instruments

X-ray viewing screen

examination room

ip stand

respirator

X-ray camera

X-ray developer

Mobile hospital units are used where emergencies might arise, such as at motor-racing circuits. This one is divided into two sections. Each has the latest equipment, so that virtually every emergency can be coped with. In the first room the patient is examined. The second room is set up as an operating theatre, so that a person brought in can be dealt with minutes after an accident.

*Above* To speed up events the rear of the emergency mobile hospital has a compressed airlift. The patient placed on the lift on a stretcher, will be raised painlessly and taken immediately for examination and, if necessary, an operation. There is a reception area where details about the patient can be taken. On the outside there are stairs, so that accompanying people do not impede the movement of the patient.

# Helping the disabled

X-rays are used for a variety of purposes. As well as showing breaks in bones (page 11) they may also show up diseases in the body, some of which affect, for example, the joints. You might know of someone who suffers from arthritis. There are two different kinds. One is called rheumatoid arthritis and the other is osteoarthritis (see diagram at the bottom of page 87). Both affect the joints, usually in the hips, the hands or the knees. It can become so bad that a person can hardly move his legs or hands at all. The extent of the disease will be shown on X-rays.

When a door squeaks, we oil the hinges to help the two parts of the mechanism to move over each other silently. The joints in our bodies are also moving for much of the time, and so they need to be lubricated. Where we have a normal joint, synovial fluid is found, which helps the bones to move easily over each other. Rheumatoid arthritis de-velops when the synovial membrane becomes inflamed and produces too much liquid. This inflammation eventually harms both the cartilage and the bone. The bone will start to wear away, and the trouble will continue until a person cannot per-form even simple actions, such as opening a door, when the fingers become affected.

Osteoarthritis is a disease which affects old people. The bones of the joints have a lining of very strong, but pliable material, called car-tilage. In later life this material often becomes brittle and breaks up. When this happens, the bones no longer move smoothly over each other. Unlike rheumatoid arthritis, however, it is still possible to move the joint, although it is very pain-ful. The amount of movement de-creases until it ceases altogether and the joint seizes up.

Scientists are constantly carrying out research to try and discover why arthritis occurs, but they have not yet been able to find a cause or to suggest why some people suffer from it and not others. In older people it is probably due to wear and tear on the joints. Sometimes it is possible to inject artificial fluid into the joints and this is often made of plastics. Nowadays surgeons can replace almost every part of the body (see page 88), including some diseased joints. During a long operation the diseased part of the bone which forms the joint is cut away. The surgeon will replace this with arti-ficial parts. He is able to do this with knee, hip and finger joints.

If you have read *Peter Pan* and *Treasure Island*, you will know that characters in these books had arti-

X-rays can be taken of various parts of the body to discover diseases at the early stages. By taking, and then studying a series of photographs it is possible to give a diagnosis of certain diseases, like osteoarthritis.

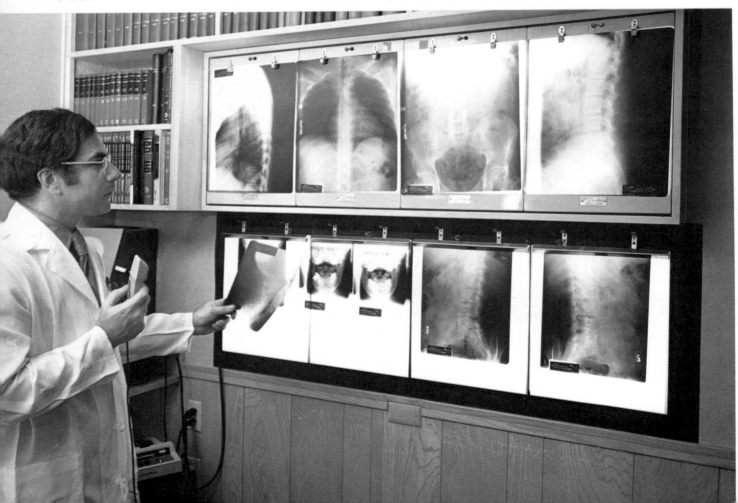

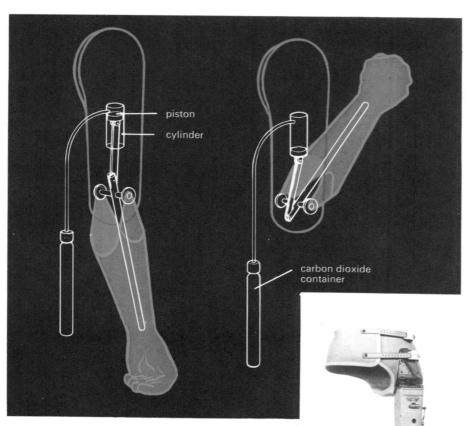

piston
cylinder

carbon dioxide
container

abled during the War that research was speeded up. Until this time the hook and the peg were the usual alternatives to real limbs.

Muscles are controlled by electrical signals which the brain sends to them. When a limb is removed, the nerves still carry impulses to the amputated end of the limb. By magnifying these, scientists have been able to use them to power artificial arms and legs. When it is not possible to do this, other methods have to be used. Pulleys can be employed and, as you will see from the diagram, carbon dioxide gas is used as a source of power to move the arm.

ficial limbs. Captain Hook took his name from the hook he had instead of a hand. Long John Silver in *Treasure Island* had a wooden leg. With modern methods it is possible to replace damaged limbs with more sophisticated devices. Much research is still going on.

Since World War II sophisticated artificial limbs have been introduced. So many people were dis-

*Above* Carbon dioxide gas is used to power this artificial arm. The gas is pushed into the cylinder, which then pushes the piston down. This operates the lever, so that the arm is pushed upwards. *Right* This artificial leg replaces one which has been removed through the hip of the patient.

*Below* In a normal knee joint *(far left)* the synovial fluid bathes the bones. When osteoarthritis occurs *(centre)*, the cartilage is destroyed and the bones of the joint rub against each other. In rheumatoid arthritis *(right)* too much fluid is made, and this causes swelling. At first the fluid damages the cartilage, and then the bone. Movement of the joint is extremely painful. It is sometimes possible to inject an artificial lubricant into the joint, which replaces any fluid which is lost, as in some types of arthritis.

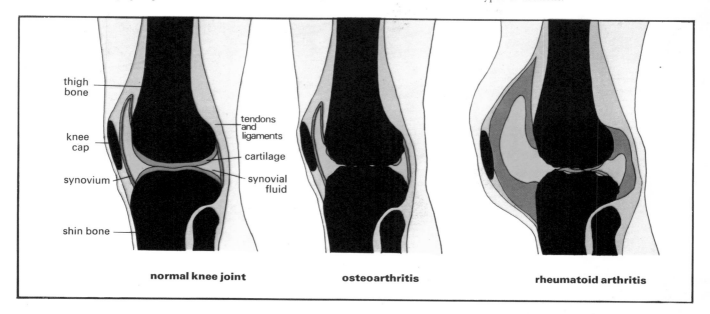

thigh bone

knee cap

synovium

shin bone

tendons and ligaments

cartilage

synovial fluid

**normal knee joint**

**osteoarthritis**

**rheumatoid arthritis**

# Spare-part surgery

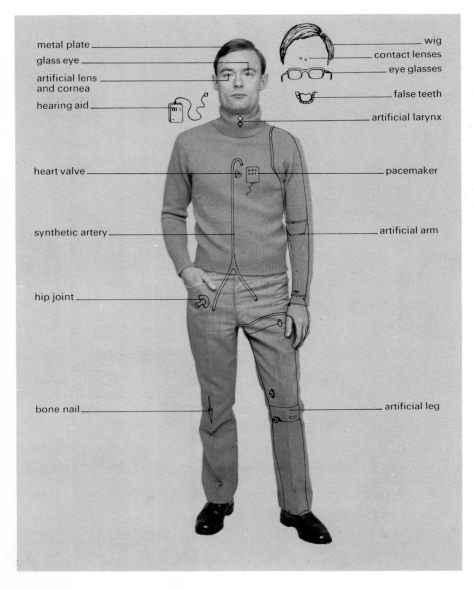

metal plate
glass eye
artificial lens and cornea
hearing aid
heart valve
synthetic artery
hip joint
bone nail

wig
contact lenses
eye glasses
false teeth
artificial larynx
pacemaker
artificial arm
artificial leg

Have a look at the illustration on this page. You can see that nearly every part of the body can be replaced through surgery by artificial pieces. Although the person shown in our picture is unlikely to have all the parts, it is quite possible for people to have more than one.

Perhaps we can't really call hearing aids, spectacles and contact lenses 'spare parts', because they don't actually become part of the body. Yet in the case of spectacles they help the lenses in the eyes to do their job much better, just as an

It is possible to replace many of the natural body parts with artificial ones. When making replacements, it is necessary to ensure that where these come into contact with existing parts of the body they will be neutral and not react against tissues and liquids.

artificial heart valve assists the person's heart.

Several parts of the eye can be replaced. It is possible to use an artificial lens – as well as contact lenses and spectacles. The transparent covering, the cornea, can also be changed. When someone has

lost an eye, an artificial one, often made of glass, will replace the missing one. Metal plates can be put into the head to replace the bone when the skull has been damaged. We have already seen how teeth can be filled if they are partly decayed. Very badly decayed ones are removed and replaced with false ones. Broken parts of teeth can sometimes be replaced.

Where deafness is only partial, a hearing aid, which is really a small amplifier, can be used. With the discovery of transistors, small hearing aids are now made. Some are so tiny that they can be concealed inside the ear; others are larger but can be hidden behind the ear.

When someone suffers from, for example, cancer of the throat, the larynx can be replaced with an artificial plastic one. Speech is still possible, although it might not be quite the same.

You will remember that the heart is a very important pump in the body. If it stops, we die, because it is no longer pumping blood round the body. We have already mentioned heart transplants. These are still quite rare operations and very complicated to perform. Other heart parts are now replaced in routine operations, but this has not always been the case. When scientists were doing research, they had to find materials which the body would not reject. The material used has to be such that it will not be affected by the body's natural defence system. For example, for damaged valves special plastic was developed, which worked very well. The tubes which the blood travels through can become diseased. When this happens, the size of the opening gets smaller, and less blood travels through them. Artificial arteries and veins can be used. These have to be made from special plastic, so that they will not be altered by the chemicals in the body.

When some joints in the body are affected by disease, they do not work efficiently; sometimes they do not work at all. These can be replaced

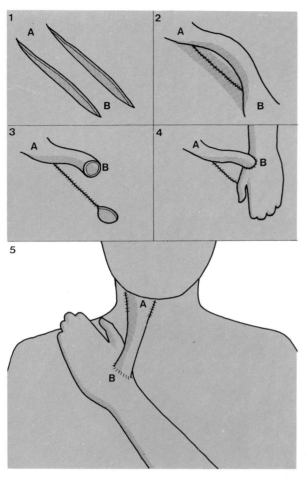

This is a pedicle graft. Cuts are made in the skin of the abdomen parallel to each other (1). 2 Shows how a tube of skin and fat is made by sewing. 3 In about six weeks one of the ends (B) is freed and then grafted (4) to a part of the patient – in this case the wrist. 5 Three weeks later the other end is freed, and this is grafted to the site where it is needed – the neck. In another three weeks the link with the wrist is cut and the excess skin taken away. Once the skin has 'taken', it will grow normally, and although there will usually be a scar, a good surgeon can make sure that this is very faint. In some people it disappears completely.

simple. When someone gets burnt, a large part of the skin may be affected. When burns have occurred, the skin has 'disappeared', and new skin has to be produced to cover the bare area. Plastic surgery can be used in such cases. It hasn't anything to do with using plastics in the repairs. The word 'plastic' in this case comes from the Greek, which means 'to shape'. This is what the surgeon does: he shapes the skin over the wound.

To shape the tissue the surgeon will often use a graft, which is a piece of skin taken from a different part of the body. He will attach the new piece of skin to the part of the body which he is treating and he will shape it to cover the area. There are several types of skin graft, and some of these are shown in the illustrations. The easiest for the surgeon to do is a free graft. He will remove a piece of skin from one part of a person's body – often a part not normally seen – and put it in the place where it is needed. If the skin is going to grow in the new area, it needs feeding, and the surgeon has to make sure that the blood supply is working.

When large areas of skin are damaged, the surgeon might have to find a donor to give some skin. If the skin comes from a different person, there may be problems. The body's defence system might reject the new skin, so that it will not grow. Careful matching of tissues has to take place before a donor is used.

with artificial joints, like those at the hips. If the whole leg is damaged, this may be removed and an artificial one attached to take its place. You will recall that if a bone normally gets broken it will repair itself (see page 11). But this does not always happen, especially when the break is a bad one, and so it may be necessary to put in a bone nail or pin to hold the broken pieces together.

Natural repairs to the body's skin are usually straightforward (see page 20). Sometimes it is not so

In burns large areas of skin are often destroyed, like the back of the hand *(top photograph)*. The surface will be carefully cleaned to get rid of disease-causing organisms. Then a layer of skin will be placed over the area. After a period of time, the exact length depending on how well the graft has taken, the area heals completely. The bottom photograph shows what can be seen after six months. You can see the join across the hand where the new skin was added.

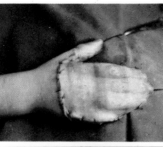

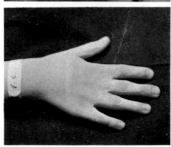

Heart valves often fail to work properly. It is now possible to replace damaged or diseased valves with plastic ones. In this example two different plastics have been used. The ring is made of polytetraflovethylene (PTFE for short). You probably know it better as the non-stick surface on a frying pan! The ball part of the valve is made of silicone rubber. Much research went on to discover the most suitable materials. Neither of those mentioned here is affected by the body, and neither causes the body to react.

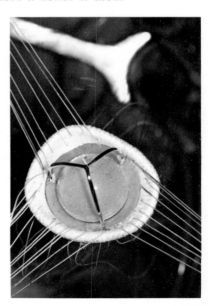

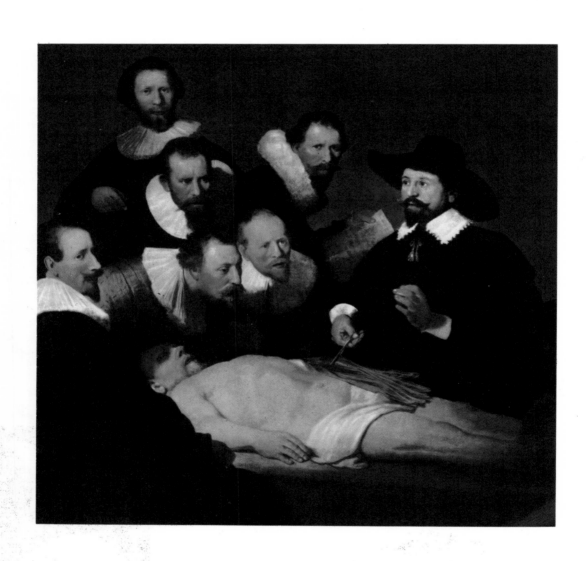

# Glossary

**Abdomen** The area of the body from the diaphragm to the pelvis. It includes the stomach, intestines, etc.

**Adolescence** The period in the growth of the body when changes take place, leading from childhood to adulthood.

**Alimentary Canal** The long tube in which the food is digested. It starts at the mouth, and includes the oesophagus, the stomach, the small and large intestines.

**Alveolus** A small air sac in the lung, in which the exchange of gases takes place. Oxygen is taken out of the air and carbon dioxide given off.

**Antibody** A substance which is made by the white blood cells. It is used by the body to deal with harmful micro-organisms, like bacteria and viruses.

**Antiseptic** A substance which attacks and breaks down the walls of bacteria (germs) and kills them. It comes from 'anti', which means against, and 'sepsis' which means decay.

**Anus** The opening at the end of the alimentary canal, through which solid waste passes out of the body.

**Anvil** One of the three small bones in the ear, named after its shape. It is the middle bone of the three ossicles–the hammer, anvil and stirrup.

**Aorta** The major blood vessel which takes the blood containing oxygen from the heart. The aorta is an artery.

**Artery** A large blood vessel with thick walls. An artery carries blood containing oxygen from the heart. All arteries, except the pulmonary artery, carry blood rich in oxygen (oxygenated blood).

**Arteriole** A small blood vessel, formed when the larger artery branches.

**Axon** The fibre part which goes out from the nerve cell. An axon carries impulses from the nerve cell.

**Bladder** A bag of tissue in which urine is stored until there is enough to be discharged by the body.

**Brain** The part within the skull which contains the nerve cells.

**Capillary** A very fine blood vessel, only wide enough to let one red blood cell move along it. The capillaries eventually join to make the arterioles.

**Carbohydrates** A food substance from which the body obtains energy. They are made up of carbon, oxygen and hydrogen. Starch, sugar and glucose are all carbohydrates.

**Carbon Dioxide** A gas in the atmosphere, some of which we breathe in. It is also removed from our bodies when we breathe out.

**Cardiac** To do with the heart, e.g. cardiac muscle, which controls the heart beat.

**Cartilage** A strong material in the body, from which part of the skeleton is made. There are discs of cartilage between the vertebrae which make up the backbone. The ends of the long bones, like the femur, are covered with this material, which gives a smooth, gliding surface, making movement easier.

**Cell** The smallest unit capable of independent life. All living things are made up of different types of cells.

**Chromosomes** Rod or thread-like structures, which occur in the nucleus of all cells. They are made up of genes, which carry the necessary information when the cell is divided. The genes also carry the messages when the sperm and ovum fuse at fertilization.

**Colon** The first and longest part of the intestine.

**Conception** The point when a male cell, the sperm, joins with the female cell, the ovum, so that a new offspring will develop.

**Cones** The cells in the retina of the eye which are sensitive to colour.

**Contraception** A means of preventing conception.

**Contraceptive** Some device, sheath, pill, etc., which is used to prevent conception–to stop the sperm and the ovum from coming together.

**Diaphragm** The wall of muscle which is between the chest and the abdomen, and is important during breathing.

**Digestion** The process, which starts in the mouth, whereby food is broken down so that it can be used by the body.

**Duodenum** The first section of the small intestine, in which digestion continues.

**Egg** The female reproductive cell–the ovum (plural ova, eggs).

**Embyro** The developing offspring growing inside the female's uterus (womb). Usually used when referring to the baby during the first four weeks after conception. After this it is known as the foetus.

**Enzyme** A chemical substance made by the body. An enzyme helps to speed up certain chemical activities in the body.

**Excretion** The process of getting rid of liquid and gaseous wastes from the body.

**Fertilization** The point at which the sperm joins with the egg.

**Foetus** A term used for a baby developing inside the uterus (womb) after the first four weeks after conception. Before this it is known as an embryo.

**Gene** A part of the chromosome which carries information to be passed on to the next generation.

**Genitals** A term used to describe the male and female reproductive organs, especially those which are outside the body.

**Haemoglobin** A pigment found in the red blood cells which increases the amount of oxygen the blood can carry.

**Hammer** One of the small bones in the ear, which resembles a hammer. The first of the three ossicles (bones)–hammer, anvil and stirrup.

**Heart** The pump which, by a series of contractions and dilations, pushes blood around the body.

**Hormone** A chemical messenger. Produced in glands in the body it is released directly into the bloodstream.

**Intestine** Part of the alimentary canal, from the lower end of the stomach to the anus. It is a long tube which is divided up into the large and small intestines. The terms large and small refer to the thickness of the tubes.

**Joint** The point at which two bones come together, so that movement can take place.

**Kidney** The organ in the body, shaped like a bean, which takes out urine from the blood. There are normally two.

**Labour** The process leading up to the birth of a baby. The first sign of activity is pain, which is brought about by muscular contractions. These are referred to as 'labour pains'.

**Ligament** The tissue which holds the bones of a joint together.

**Liver** A large organ which performs a number of very important jobs in the body, including the purification of the blood. It also secretes bile.

**Lung** A muscular bag made up of small air sacs (alveoli) and air passages. Oxygen is taken out of the air which we breathe in, and carbon dioxide and other waste gases discharged, and breathed out.

**Lymph** A liquid, not unlike blood, but without the cells. It bathes the body cells.

**Lymphocyte** One type of white cell, which is responsible for making antibodies.

**Mitochondria** Called the 'powerhouse of the cell', each mitochondrion is very small, and is concerned with the release of energy.

**Muscle** A collection of cells which can contract and relax, so that movement can take place.

**Nerve** A thin fibre which carries messages between the body and the brain or spinal cord, and vice versa.

**Neuron** The nerve cell.

**Nucleus** The central part of every living cell, which controls the activities and contains the chromosomes, which are made up of genes.

**Oesophagus** A tube which starts at the mouth and goes to the stomach, along which food passes.

**Ossicles** The three small bones in the ear – the hammer, anvil and stirrup.

**Ovary** The female reproductive organ, in which the ova (eggs) are stored. From puberty until the menopause one egg is usually released each month from alternative ovaries. There are two ovaries in the body, and eggs are not released during pregnancy.

**Oxygen** A gas in the atmosphere which is taken out of the air by the lungs. It is needed by every living cell during the process of respiration.

**Penis** The male organ, through which sperm is released. Urine is also discharged through the penis.

**Peristalsis** Muscular contractions of the alimentary canal, which help to move food along.

**Phagocytes** White blood cells which are able to help protect the body from infection by dealing with bacteria.

**Placenta** The tissues which develop in the female's womb when she becomes pregnant, and present a 'barrier' between the mother and child. It allows food to pass to the embryo/foetus, and waste products to be eliminated.

**Plasma** The liquid part of the blood, without the cells. The white and red corpuscles and the platelets float in this liquid.

**Puberty** The stage during adolscence when sexual characteristics develop in the body, making reproduction possible.

**Rectum** The last part of the large intestine, which finishes at the anus.

**Renal** To do with the kidneys, e.g. renal artery.

**Reproduction** The process in which ovum and sperm will join together, to start a new life.

**Respiration** A complicated process in which oxygen is used by body cells, so that energy is released from food substances.

**Rods** The cells in the retina of the eye which detect light intensity.

**Sperm** The male reproductive cells. Sperms are produced in the testes.

**Spinal Cord** The long nerve which is found inside the spinal column.

**Spine** The backbone or vertebral column, which is made up of small bones, the vertebrae.

**Stirrup** One of the small bones in the ear. It gets its name from its shape. It is the third of three ossicles – hammer, anvil and stirrup.

**Stomach** The muscular bag in which food collects. It is here that the main part of digestion takes place.

**Tendon** A piece of tissue by which the end of a muscle is attached to a bone.

**Testes** The male reproductive organs in which the sperms are made. The testes hang outside the body between the legs of the male, in a sac of skin called the scrotum.

**Tissue** A collection of cells of the same sort, which make up all or part of an organ.

**Tonsils** Glands situated in the throat. They produce large numbers of white cells, and help to trap and destroy bacteria.

**Umbilical Cord** The tube which attaches the foetus/embryo to the placenta, which in turn connects it with the female.

**Uterus** The part of the female reproductive system in which the embryo/foetus develops: it is often called the womb.

**Vagina** The part of the female reproductive system from the uterus to the outside. The baby is born through this passage.

**Vein** The blood tubes in the body which, with the exception of the pulmonary vein, carries blood from which most of the oxygen has been removed (deoxygenated blood).

**Venule** The small branch of a vein. A tube which carries blood which has been to the cells of the body.

**Vertebral** A small bone, a number of which make up the vertebral or spinal column.

**Vertebral Column** See Spine.

**Womb** See Uterus.

**Zygote** The cell produced when the sperm and the egg join together at fertilization.

# Index

The figures in *italics* refer to illustrations and those in **bold** letters indicate an entry in the Glossary (pages 91–2).

# Acknowledgments

The author and publisher would like to thank those who have given their permission for illustrations to be reproduced in this book. All diagrams are reproduced by permission of Orbis Publishing Limited unless otherwise credited. The diagrams on pages 49, 62, 63, 64, 67, 69*tr*, 71 were prepared by Lorraine Richardson.

Aldus Books 89*br* (Edwards Laboratories Inc., Santa Ana, California)

Armstrong, Dr P. 22

Aspect 57*tl*

Bavestrelli, Bevilacqua and Prato 51*b*

Bevilacqua, C. 8, 11*br*

Bibliothèque Laurentienne 82*t*

Boardman, Ron 20*tl*, 35 *t*

Brierley, Paul 70*b*

Camera Press 3, 61*t*, 68 (Bachrach)

Caprotti, Gio 11*tr*, 21*c*

Castano, P. 21, 33*r*, 52, 74, 75*bl*

Marshall Cavendish 51*t* (John Watney), 59*c*, 59*b* (J. J. Mollitt)

Ciccione, C. 80

Colorific 28*bl* (Terence Le Goubin), 43*b*

Cranham 26*bl* (Rapho)

Daily Telegraph 73*r*

Dickins, Douglas 57*c*

Euro Colour Library 62*br*

Mary Evans Picture Library 39*t*

Fox Photos 43*t*

IBM 55

IGDA 8, 9, 13*tl*, 14*b*, 19, 28*br*, 30, 31, 35*b*, 40, 46, 47, 57*br*, 59*t*, 60, 65, 69*l*, 70*t*, 73*l*, 75*t*, 77*c*, 79*tr*, 87, 88, 89*bl*, 90

Keystone Press 61*b*, 86

King's College Hospital 71*t*

Lalance 79*t*

Leeds Royal Infirmary 11*tl*

Mansell Collection 78, 79*bl*, 81*bl*

Martini, P. 41*b*, 75*bl*

Museo di Storia delle Scienze, Leida 79*br* (F. Arborio Mella)

Orbis 18, 21*t* and 21*bl* (John Watney), 27*t* (Le Goubin), 28*t* (Ray Dean) 41*t* and 82*b* (Derek Bayes)

Picturepoint 83

Radio Times Hulton Picture Library 81*t*

Ronan Picture Library 81*br*

Royal Postgraduate Medical School 20*br* (Dr S. M. Lewis)

Spectrum Colour Library 16*l*

Sunday Times 81*c*, 85*t*

University of Minnesota 37*t*

UPI 84*t*

Watney, John 46*bl*

Yoga World 13*tr*